MUSHROOM MANIA

Hilary E. Bartlett

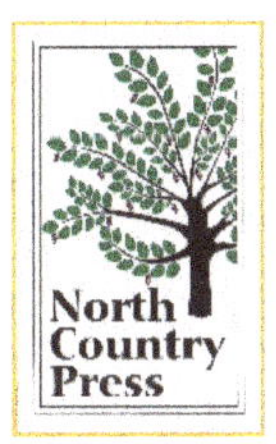

MUSHROOM MANIA

Cover design, Linda Sapienza

Artwork, Hilary Bartlett

ISBN 978-1-943424-81-8

LCCN 2023942273

North Country Press
Unity, ME 04988

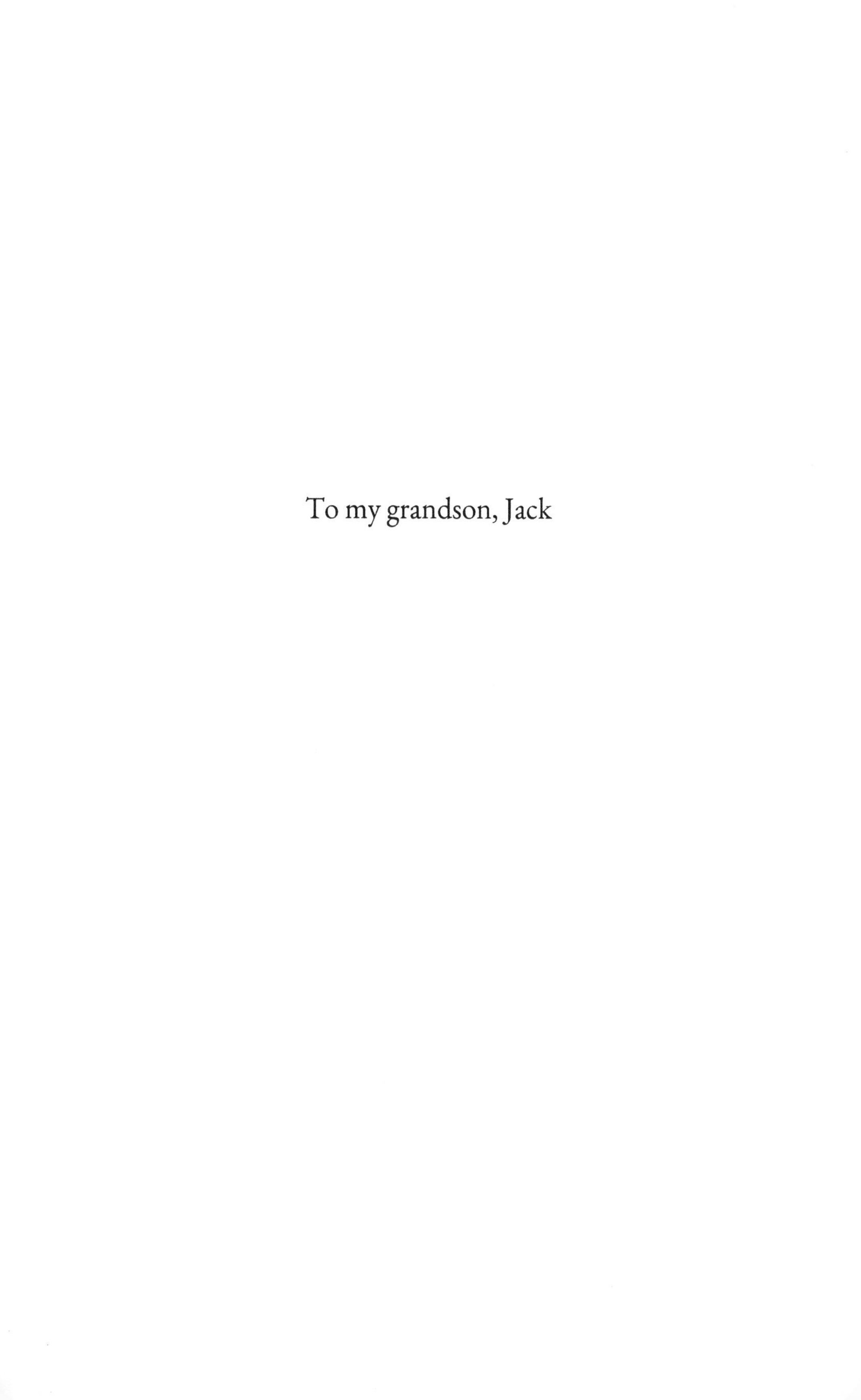

To my grandson, Jack

TABLE OF CONTENTS

Mushrooms

Overnight, very
Whitely, discreetly,
Very quietly

Our toes, our noses
Take hold on the loam,
Acquire the air.

Nobody sees us,
Stops us, betrays us;
The small grains make room.

Soft fists insist on
Heaving the needles,
The leafy bedding,

Even the paving.
Our hammers, our rams,
Earless and eyeless,

Perfectly voiceless,
Widen the crannies,
Shoulder through holes. We

Diet on water,
On crumbs of shadow,
Bland-mannered, asking

Little or nothing.
So many of us!
So many of us!

We are shelves we are
Tables, we are meek,
We are edible,

Nudgers and shovers
In spite of ourselves.
Our kind multiplies:

We shall by morning
Inherit the earth.
Our foot's in the door.

—Sylvia Plath

INTRODUCTION

Mushrooms are having their moment — sales have soared. While white buttons are still popular, Maine growers have pumped up production of more fresh varieties to meet increased demand at restaurants, farmers markets and grocery stores. More individuals also hit the woods to forage wild ones. In spring, crowds flocked to Maine Mushroom Fest to munch on mushrooms, learn about their healing powers and how to grow edible species at home. *Edible Maine* magazine has referred to our state as 'Shroom Nation'.

Mushrooms are visible fruit bodies of hidden fungi that weave intricate webs of feeding tubes through wood and soil. A mushroom's sole purpose in life is reproduction. It sheds masses of spores that enable a fungus to multiply. Mushrooms disperse spores like plants disperse seeds — floating on water and wind or hitchhiking on bodies of insects and animals. We notice spores only as smoky clouds released from puffballs or as a fine dust that settles on surfaces. To see spores in more detail we would need a microscope.

Maine's woodlands and forests are carpeted with mushrooms in soft bride-like hues, bright lipstick reds or lavender blues, plus subtle greens and every conceivable shade of yellow and brown. Short-lived fleshy ones with flat or bell-shaped caps on stalks resemble miniature pedestal tables or umbrellas. Some mushroom caps grow as large as dinner plates, others are as small as a dime. Tough fan-shaped shelves or hoof-shaped mushrooms—commonly referred to as conks—develop on trees or downed logs. You may come across mushrooms disguised as balls, cups, sea corals and starfish. Others resemble cauliflowers or bird-like nests with clutches of eggs. Convoluted, rubbery or jellied forms stiffen and contract when dry. Firm tuberous truffles shelter underground and withstand drought.

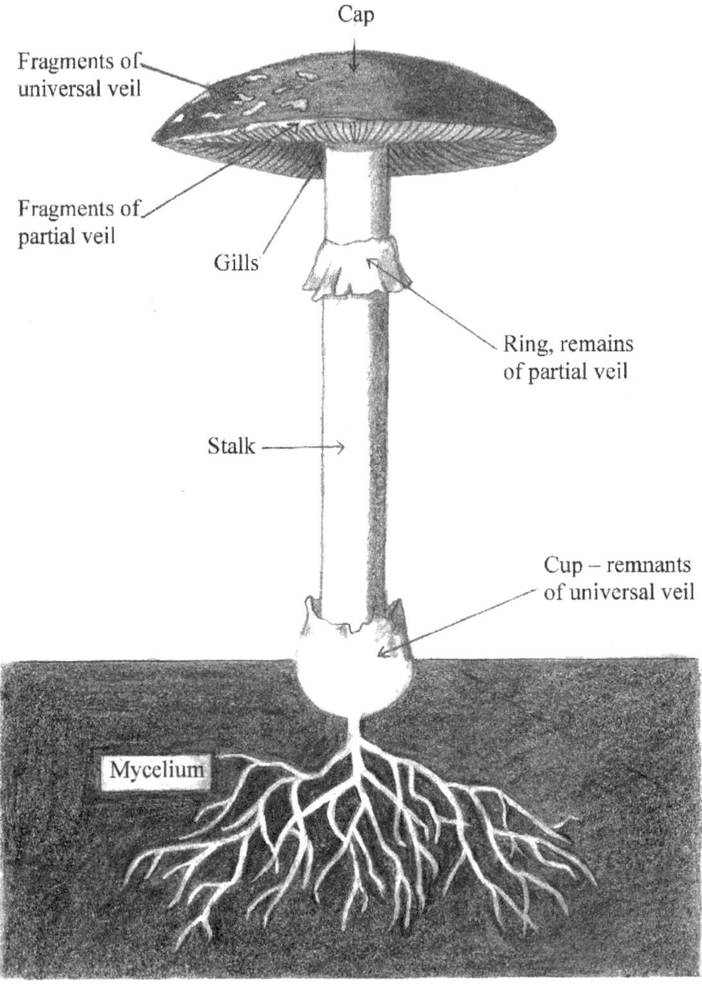

Parts of a gilled cap mushroom. The entire structure is the fruit body of a fungus.

For thousands of years, mushrooms have been foraged for food and healing in various parts of the world. At least 350 species are edible and about 700 have verified therapeutic value.

Ancient Greeks harvested agarikon (a hefty tree mushroom) to prolong life. According to Greek mythology, the god Zeus sent a lightning bolt down to Earth to create mushrooms that would give strength to warriors. Zeus's son, Perseus, drank water from a mushroom at a site he named Mycenae during his journey to slay the monstrous Medusa with living snakes for hair. The term mycology (the study of fungi) was derived from the Greek, mykes = mushroom + logos = discourse.

On a recent visit to Egypt I learned that pharaohs decreed mushrooms were sacred plants of immortality reserved for royalty, gifts from the god Osiris. Commoners were forbidden to eat or even touch them. My mouth dropped as our Egyptian guide, Ishmael, led us through temples where mushroom-shaped pillars reached to the sky. Ishmael translated hieroglyphs and pointed out images of mushrooms carved on sandstone walls.

Painted Chinese characters on archaic parchment scrolls describe the many medicinal properties of mushrooms. Taoist and Buddhist physicians pressed mushrooms (good-omen food) into the hands of their patients. Healing lingzhi, translated as divine mushroom, grow on the steep slopes of China's sacred mountains. These mushrooms resemble red lacquered fans. A Chinese text from 206 BCE prescribes lingzhi mushrooms for longevity. References to lingzhi appeared in a fundamental religious text of Taoism, the *Tao Te Ching*. Lingzhi mushrooms were a popular motif in ancient Chinese art, often portrayed in a hand of a wise sage or renowned scholar. Lingzhi are known as reishi in Japan, but for longevity Japanese people swear by shiitake mushrooms. In Japan's feudal era, shiitake were reserved for lords but some peasants took their chances and foraged the forbidden mushrooms. Maitake mushrooms were prized for their curative powers. Daimyo noblemen traded them for their weight in silver from a shōgun (military leader). Japanese families fiercely guarded locations of their maitake trees, the secret revealed only by an elder on his deathbed to his oldest or favorite son.

People have hunted and gathered mushrooms for centuries in Europe. Wild mushrooms traditionally provided nourishment when crops failed. Russian mushroom lore is passed down to younger generations through poems and songs that teach children the names of common wild varieties. In the Russian nursery rhyme, *Panic Amongst the Mushrooms*, the main character, Borovik (a peppery milk cap), tries but fails to enlist others to join his army as different types of mushrooms march through the stanzas.

In the Americas, shamans of indigenous tribes bowed to the agarikon mushroom's sacred health-giving properties. Yet early American settlers shuddered and wrinkled their noses at mushrooms. British immigrants reviled them as toadstools associated with poison and decay. Most newcomers from Eastern Europe cast off their parents' mushroom lore to fit in with their new country. This has changed.

The earliest record of mushroom cultivation (1209 CE) was of shiitake in China's Song dynasty. Louis XIV's gardener cultivated our now common, white, button mushrooms from a wild variety. He nurtured them on compost in open fields at Versailles. French Emperor and military leader, Napoleon, moved mushroom production into damp limestone caves under Paris where they sprouted on heaps of horse dung, a readily available resource. Nowadays, white button mushrooms are farmed all over the world because this variety shoots up fast with high yields on cheap agricultural waste. Customers also clamor for baby bellas and portabellas (the same species as white buttons) because their taste and texture are similar to meat.

Aztec and Mayan civilizations (BCE) used a variety of hallucinogenic mushrooms as mediators in religious ceremonies. The term 'magic mushrooms' first appeared in a 1956 *Life* magazine article about indigenous Mexican tribes who ate hallucinogenic mushrooms during sacred rituals.

Mushroom magic threads through British folktales in part because of mushroom circles known as fairy rings. They form after wet weather in late summer to early fall. Legends claim that fairies danced in them. Prospero in Shakespeare's play, *The Tempest*, alludes to a superstition that sheep balk at eating grass in fairy rings. In many European regions mushroom circles symbolized sorcery — places where witches cast spells and gnomes buried treasure. Peasants quaked with fear when they came across a mushroom ring and refused to enter it.

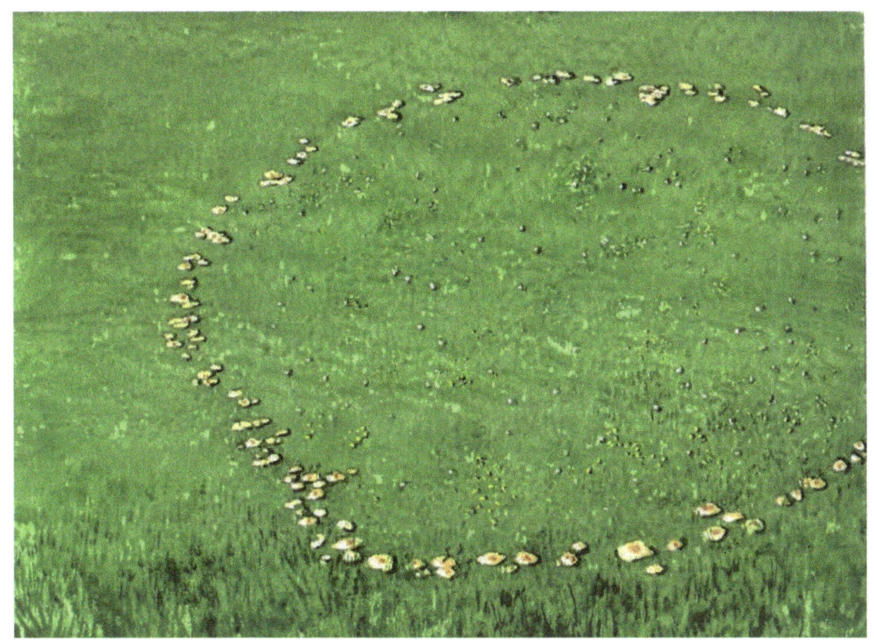

Mushroom fairy ring.

Shamans in the Baltic States and Russia visited spirit worlds by eating hallucinogenic fly agaric mushrooms. This species, with its bright red cap and white spots, is woven throughout centuries of European folktales. Can reindeer really fly or did the legend arise from Saami herdsmen of Lapland and Siberia? They fed fly agaric mushrooms to reindeer then collected their urine from snow to make a hallucinogenic (but detoxified) beverage. Santa's suit may symbolize red deer pelts worn by herders, but a more intriguing theory is that Santa's red and white costume mimics colors of the fly agaric mushroom.

Images of the fly agaric skitter across fantastical childhood stories that endure. An imperious caterpillar in Lewis Caroll's Wonderland tempts Alice to eat some of his mushroom, an offer she accepts which results in her neck stretching as long as a serpent. In 1967, Jefferson Airplane belted out the band's lyrics to *White Rabbit* at the Monterey Pop Festival:

"And you've just had some kind of mushroom
And your mind is moving low.
Go ask Alice
I think she'll know."

Mushroom-inspired images swirled over sleeves of rock albums and posters during the 1960s hippie scene, an era that blossomed with psychedelic imagery and 'shroom'-induced mind-blowing experiences.

Mushrooms popped up in earlier pop culture, perhaps the most famous in *Fantasia*, the Disney feature film released in 1940 that coupled symphonic musical themes with cartoon animations. Trills of a flute and notes from plucked strings accompanied mushrooms that jumped and scurried across a screen to Tchaikovsky's Chinese Dance from *The Nutcracker*. The jaunty fungi even made the album cover of the score, performed by Leopold Stokowski and the Philadelphia Orchestra.

The charm of mushroom animation continued. Characters called Smurfs debuted in a 1950s Belgian comic series. They made their teeny forest homes from hollowed out mushrooms that suited the Smurfs' distinct personalities. The tiny blue humanoids starred in an animated 1980s TV show. During the same decade, a Nintendo video game, *Super Mario*, featured mushroom people whose contact with Mario or his brother, Luigi, made the two heroes larger and more powerful. The mushroom people were fundamental to all the games in the Mario series and arguably the most important magical helpers.

Fungi (molds, yeasts and mushrooms) appear in fossil records from over one billion years ago.

An eighteenth-century scientist, Linnaeus, divided all living things into plants or animals. Within my lifetime, fungi have been placed in a separate kingdom on the Tree of Life, closer to animals than plants.

Miss Kate Furbish described and painted about 500 mushrooms in her extensive study of Maine flora (1870 – 1908), because in her day mushrooms were still regarded as plants. The intrepid lady botanist travelled by stagecoach down to York and up to Aroostook counties to collect a wide range of specimens. Wild mushrooms poked their heads from her basket as she tramped through meadows, woodlands, forests and valleys or clambered over hills and river banks. Miss Furbish gifted her life-work to Bowdoin College in the Maine town where she had made her home.

The dawn of molecular biology in the 1950s and subsequent DNA analyses upended mushroom classification. Prior to that they were grouped by what they looked like, where they grew, how they released spores and whether they helped or hurt trees. Over 1.5 million fungi have been identified, approximately 10% produce mushrooms. New fungal species are found every day at a rate of about 2,000 per year. Many of the world's mushrooms also remain undiscovered.

Advantages

Fungi play a key role as Nature's housekeepers, they sustain us as either food or medicine, and we use them in wide a range of industrial applications.

Decomposition and nutrient cycling — Fungi break down complex, dead, organic waste material into simple accessible nutrients for living organisms.

Support of crop and forest health — Fungal associations with plant roots benefit the plant hosts.

Soil maintenance — Mycelium (a vast fungal network of feeding tubes) binds soil particles and prevents fertile land from turning into desert.

Food — Edible mushrooms are low in calories and unhealthy saturated fats, yet loaded with antioxidants, vitamins and minerals. Blue molds ripen and add flavor to cheese. Yeast fermentation causes bread to rise and produces alcoholic beverages.

Economic growth — Maine's mushroom industry supplies jobs and adds revenue to the state.

Scientific research — Because we share many genes with fungi, research on these organisms has led to insights on human aging and how coding errors cause disease.

Healing mushrooms — Some fungi contain compounds that strengthen human immune systems and prevent degenerative diseases.

Antibiotics — Fungi make chemicals that destroy or inhibit growth of microorganisms that cause disease.

Other pharmaceuticals — Genetically-modified yeasts produce vitamins, insulin and therapeutic proteins. One mold synthesizes gestodene, an active ingredient of contraceptive pills. Fungal cyclosporine is an immunosuppressant used for transplant patients.

Pesticides — Some fungi ward off or destroy insects.

Manufacturing — Digestive fungal enzymes speed up chemical reactions at room temperature to make paper, process cotton and convert corn starch into high fructose syrup.

Environmental cleaners — White rot fungi degrade toxic chemicals into harmless substances.

Sustainable construction materials — A few fungi convert man-made plastics into biodegradable material for building blocks.

Biodegradable fungal products, a substitute for man-made polymers — Mycelium-based material is replacing plastic dashboard car-parts, Styrofoam™ packaging, polyurethane acoustic panels and foam furniture, as well as petroleum-based faux leather.

Mushroom dyes — Mushroom pigments make colorfast nonpolluting dyes for textiles, paper and wood.

Mushroom Batteries — Mushrooms are an inexpensive eco-friendly alternative for graphite anodes currently used in lithium batteries. Plus a higher porosity of mushroom tissue provides more potential for energy storage.

Biofuels — Oil in fungal cells is a potential biofuel. Fungal enzymes convert crop waste into sugars that are fermented by yeast into ethanol, a gasoline additive.

Disadvantages

We reap many benefits from fungi yet they also cause excessive damage. Although some mushrooms may save your life, others make you sick.

Toxic mushrooms — A number of mushroom varieties are poisonous; most are non-lethal but a few are deadly.

Food Spoilage — Molds attack fresh produce and even spoil food in your fridge. Other fungi tolerate high sugar levels used to preserve jams, jellies and syrups.

Material damage — Mycelium growth ruins furniture, leather, fabric, marble and granite. Fungi attack wooden fences, telephone poles, railroad ties, wood-framed houses and pit props used in mines.

Accumulation of toxic chemicals — Mushrooms concentrate harmful chemicals from polluted land, air and water, which means we have to closely monitor our food supply.

Disease — A number of fungal species act as pathogens that kill host cells then feed on the dead organic material.

Fungal ringworm erupts on human skin to form scaly, red, circular lesions. The fungus may discolor nails, travel down to infect hair follicles, or even snuggle up in warm moist crannies between our toes. Dust-like fungal spores may cause asthma attacks or allergic reactions. Sensitivity increases with continued exposure. Mushroom farmers wear face masks to prevent breathing in high concentrations of spores — fungi seize a foothold when given an opportunity. Some cause lung disease, others enter a bloodstream and circulate to infect the whole body.

Fungal white nose syndrome of bats has rapidly spread throughout America over the last decade, drastically reducing population size.

Predatory fungi capture nematode worms in sticky mycelium nets, or paralyze them with toxins in order for fungal threads to infiltrate worm bodies and digest them. A zombie fungus infects carpenter ants then changes ant behavior with mind-altering chemicals that help the fungus multiply. A mushroom sprouts from an ant's head and sheds spores, while mycelium grows inside an insect's body until it explodes. This sinister strategy by a zombie fungus was used for the plot of a novel, *The Girl with All the Gifts*.

Fungal mildews, rusts, smuts and wilts threaten global food security. They sneak up and leave acres of decimated crops in their wake. Millions of civilians and legions of soldiers throughout the Roman Empire died from a fungus that formed toxic resting bodies in rye husks used for bread. Peasants in the Middle Ages bent their knees and prayed when outbreaks of this crop parasite took hold in the hope that God would remove the blight if they repented for their sins.

In the early 1900s, flare-ups of fungal rusts swept across the grain belt and Indian plains of America, covering crops with rust-colored pustules. Further losses were thwarted in the 1960s by breeding resistant strains of wheat.

Increased global trade and travel has led to a worldwide increase of fungal plant diseases. Spores land on travelers' clothes, freight or produce and are transported to other countries. New fungal pathogens emerge, which jump to foreign hosts and flourish in different geographic locations.

Aspects of fungal blights are being studied at the University of Maine by Dr. Seanna Annis, who conducts research on fungi that cause disease of lowbush blueberries; fungal pathogens are identified by Dr. Alicyn Smart at a plant disease diagnostic lab.

Spores gain access to sapwood after bears and deer rip off bark or woodpeckers drill holes with their beaks. Discolored leaves, deformed tree limbs and cankers signal a fungal attack. Giant chestnuts along the east coast of the United States have virtually disappeared — blighted by a fungus. Yellowed wilted leaves in the 1970s heralded the arrival of Dutch elm disease in several Maine towns. Fungal spores had hitched a ride on bodies of wood-boring beetles. Many old-timers still reminisce about the leafy canopied elms that once lined both sides of Main Street in Thomaston. Back then, black oily creosote hugged wooden telephone poles to ward off fungal growth.

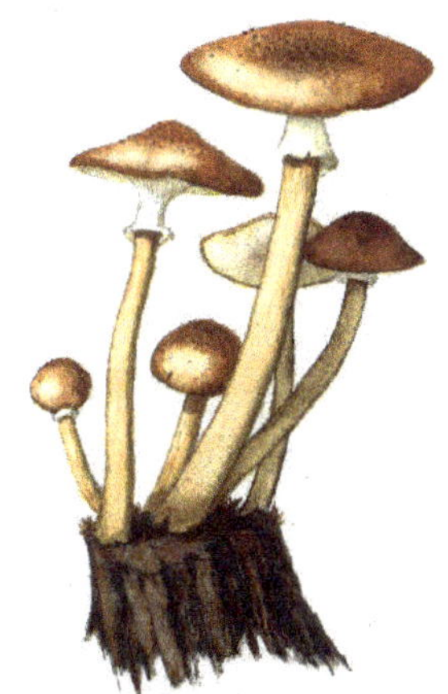

Honey mushroom, *Armillaria mellea*

The clever honey fungus survives by aggressively switching from parasite to decomposer mode in order to feed its voracious appetite. And this strategy is enormously successful. One honey fungus in the Blue Mountains of Oregon stretches for six square miles. Carbon dating puts this fungus at over 2,000 years old, DNA analysis revealed it is a giant clone. Honey mushrooms spring up from a central base, the only visible sign of this massive, subterranean, feeding machine. Named for their color as opposed to their taste, you may also find honey mushrooms in woodlands throughout Maine. At night, their mycelium gives off a dim blue-green light commonly referred to as foxfire.

———————

I consume mushrooms, in turn they have consumed much of my life. My introduction to mycology was as a technician at J. Bibby and Sons' research lab in Liverpool, England. I investigated the effectiveness of fungal enzymes to remove stubborn stains in order to improve Bibby's laundry detergent. Fan-shaped appendages bearing fungal spores also waved at me when I peered down a microscope at audacious molds that resisted fungicides. I eventually left Bibby's to study mycology at university, where I obtained a degree in microbiology. My passion for mushrooms flourished as I tossed them in untried recipes and shot photos of wild varieties when I first moved to rural Maine. I stumbled upon a dapple-lit wonderland, Oven's Mouth in Boothbay, where mushrooms poked through moss and leaf litter along steep banks of a tidal waterway.

Perhaps mushrooms will impact your life as well?

———————

This book is not meant to be a scientific discourse but aims to introduce nature-lovers, foodies and health-conscious souls to the fascinating world of mushrooms. An extensive bibliography is provided for those who seek more details.

HOW FUNGI FUNCTION

What They Eat

Fungi feast on dead things.

Each fungus toils as a massive feeding body, a mycelium made up of miniscule interconnected tubes that suck energy out of organic waste. As long as fungi have food and water they will thrive. Mycelium resembles a mat of tangled cotton threads to our eyes. It branches and burrows through soil, one cubic inch may contain up to eight miles of mycelium. Dried out mycelium slumbers, but wakes up when doused with water.

Fungi act as recyclers. Their digestion converts large, complex, organic molecules of dead carcasses, plants and trees into small, simple, accessible nutrients for living organisms. Acids and enzymes ooze out of microscopic fungal tubes called hyphae in order to convert organic waste into soluble nutrients.

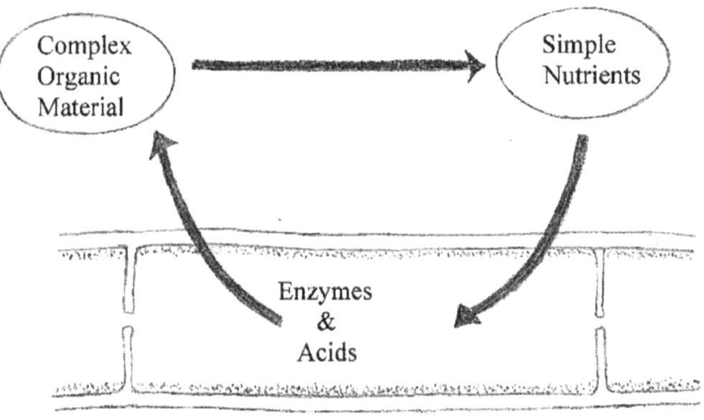

Flow of enzymes, acids and digested soluble nutrients in and out of hyphae. Central pores in cross walls allow chemical transport through mycelium.

These are absorbed back into hyphae and channeled to other parts of a mycelium for growth, repair and mushroom production. Nourished mycelium rapidly spreads. New territory is readily conquered because fungi can morph into unique strains that gobble up foreign substances. Soil is formed from fungal byproducts, their enzymes make humus and their acids mineralize rock. Hyphae release a sticky glue that binds soil particles, which prevents erosion. Prolonged drought kills off mycelium — soil blows away.

A microscale bacterial community functions outside fungal cell walls. This microbiome benefits fungal health and enables a mycelium to conquer large habitats. Everything within an ecosystem is connected, one group depends upon another.

Mushroom circles (fairy rings) form when central mycelium dies after food in soil runs out. Some circles are as wide as a coffee table, others are as wide as a Ferris wheel. A brown dead zone sometimes forms within lawn rings or a central, lush, green patch of new grass springs up after a nutrient spike when old mycelium dies. Scotch bonnets (fairy ring mushrooms) crop up on lawns and meadows during fall in Maine. They endure drought and rehydrate when moisture returns to produce new spores. Mushroom circles also spread on forest floors, growing radially by three to five inches each year.

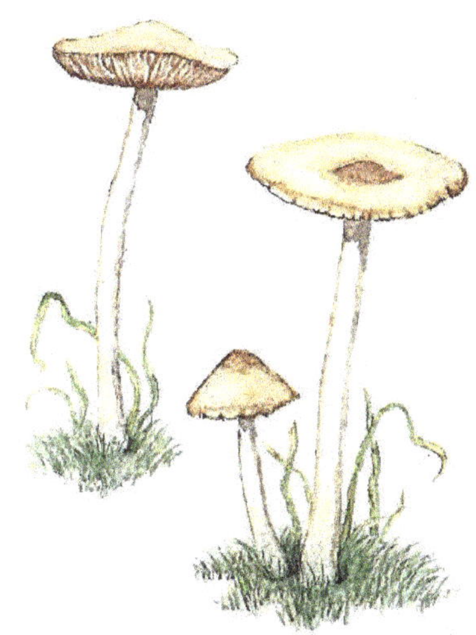

Scotch bonnet (fairy ring mushroom), *Marasmius oreades.*

White rot fungi devour lignin, the tough woody tissue of trees. Fungal peroxidase enzymes crack apart the close-knit chemical bonds of lignin into simple glucose molecules. This results in pale bleached wood. Apart from a few bacterial species, other decomposers (worms, slugs and snails) are unable to break down woody lignin. Some fungi munch on plant cellulose which causes brown rot of trees.

Without fungal decomposers our forests would choke and we would have to wade through piles of debris miles deep.

Table 1. Fungi that Cause Wood Rot of Maine Trees. All of these fungi produce mushrooms.

Fungi	**White rot** **Breaks down lignin**	**Brown rot** **Breaks down cellulose**
Oyster mushrooms	+	
Angel wings	+	
Turkey tail	+	
Tinder conk	+	
Artist's conk	+	
Reishi	+	
Maitake	+	
Chaga	+	
Lion's mane	+	
Honey mushrooms	+	
Split-gill mushrooms	+	
Dryad's saddle	+	
Birch polypore		+
Chicken-of-the-woods		+
Red-belted polypore		+

Ostry et al. 2011.
Stamets 2005.
www.mushroomexpert.com

Fungi are first in line to colonize a garbage dump. A waste pile shrinks over time because fungi convert most of the biomass into carbon dioxide and water. A secondary wave of bacteria, insects, slugs and worms gobble up organic leftovers.

Certain fungal species make special digestive juices that chew through man-made polymers and toxic substances. Fungi might be one answer to reduce plastic waste. We applauded the invention of plastic as a godsend, but because of its durability we now face a massive pollution problem. Most bacteria are unable to degrade man-made plastics and resins. White-rot fungi can break them down because they produce enzymes that dismantle strong chemical bonds of lignin (a complex polymer that makes trees rigid and woody). In 2017, scientists isolated a polyurethane-eating mold from a landfill in Pakistan. Architects and interior designers chasing down biodegradable components latched onto this idea. They coaxed a fungus to change discarded plastic into structural building blocks. Since then, fifty more plastic-eating fungi have been discovered.

We currently bury or burn toxic waste, yet fungi can clean up polluted sites. Some species degrade pesticides, explosives and dangerous compounds in electrical equipment or preservatives. Other fungi dismantle chemical bonds of nerve toxins or adapt to use a contaminant as their sole food source. Shiitake and oyster mushrooms magically decolorize dyes from industrial effluent. Enzymes of turkey tail and oyster mushrooms convert harmful hydrocarbons of coal, crude oil and petroleum into smaller less noxious molecules. In one field trial, oyster mushrooms cleaned up gasoline and diesel in contaminated soil at less cost than other methods (incineration, solvent extraction, solidification, venting, washing and indirect thermal). A variety of fungi absorb toxic heavy-metals. Mushrooms accumulate more than mycelium. Oyster mushrooms stock-pile mercury up to 145 times above background levels. Mycoremediation projects often use shaggy mane ink caps because they readily leach out cadmium, arsenic and mercury.

Table 2. Fungal Cleaners of Pollutants. All of these fungi produce mushrooms.

Fungus	Contaminants
Turkey tail	PAHs, TNT, organophosphates, mercury
Shaggy mane	Arsenic, mercury, cadmium
Pearl oyster mushroom	PAHs, PCBs, cadmium, mercury, dioxins
Shiitake	PAHs, PCBs, PCPs

PCBs – polychlorinated biphenyls in electrical equipment and carbonless copy paper.
PAHs – polycyclic aromatic hydrocarbons in crude oil, gasoline and creosote wood preservative.
PCPs – pentachorophenols in pesticides and wood preservatives.
TNT – trinitrotoluene in explosives.
Stamets 2019.

Dense blocks of fungal mycelium trap silt and bacterial pathogens, such as *E. coli,* from polluted water — a possible low-tech solution to clean up effluent from Maine farms. Breathable burlap bags of mycelium stacked side by side at a boundary of a watershed reduce contaminants in surface flow, plus burlap fabric is decomposable. Mycelium filtration barriers with multiple organisms may be needed to detoxify sites with a complex mix of pollutants.

A number of factory assembly lines have 'gone green' and churn out car parts made from fungal itaconic acid instead of synthetic rubber or plastic. Your kids may soon be building LEGO® structures with itaconic fungal bricks.

The mycelium produced by fungal degradation of waste material is also an eco-friendly choice for many different materials including building insulation and a substitute for polyurethane foam currently used for furniture. Ikea and Dell have already switched from Styrofoam™ to mycelium packaging to ship their goods. Sound engineering has also jumped into mycelium-based acoustic panels and 3D printed earplugs. Evocative Design, in upper New York State, produces a squishy fungal-based foam that has better insulating qualities than polystyrene. The company also makes bricks, tiles, particle board and lamps as well as faux leather from mycelium. Bolt Threads produces a mycelium-based leather called Mylo™ in the Netherlands. In March of 2021, Stella McCartney launched a new garment line in the U.K. made from this fungal fabric. Models strutted down a catwalk in black Mylo™ bustiers and utility pants. Stella stated that her mycelium-derived material had a much lower carbon footprint than petroleum-based faux leather and calf hide. Adidas swiftly followed with a Stan Smith Mylo™ brand white shoe. MycoWorks, in California, manipulate reishi growth to make a leather-like material (Fine Mycelium™) that is supple, soft, and strong.

Partnerships with Plants

Ninety percent of plants share a cozy nutritional relationship with fungi. Plant roots release a sticky goo that attracts fungal hyphae. They hug root hairs to form an underground mycorrhiza (*myco* = fungus, *rhizal* = root) that benefits both partners. Masses of fine mycelium tendrils provide a greater surface area to sop up more water than plant roots. Mycorrhizal fungi scavenge soil for water, nitrogen and minerals, which they trade for sugars produced by plant photosynthesis. A plant may provide 30% of a fungus's carbon requirement. Mycorrhizal fungi leach out low concentrations of nutrients in harsh heathlands and tundra, which helps their plant hosts. Fungi supply 80% of a plant's nitrogen demand and up to 100% of its phosphorus, elements vital for growth. Plants were able to colonize continents only because their mycorrhizal fungi mined for minerals. Fossils of mycorrhiza have been discovered in rocks over 500 million years old.

One mycelium may have mycorrhiza with several trees. One tree may have mycorrhiza with several fungi. Mushrooms such as king boletes, black trumpets, morels, maitake, hedgehogs, milk caps and matsutake sprout near specific types of trees because of mycorrhizal associations. Some edible mushrooms defy cultivation because their growth depends on living plants. Fungal partnerships with roots strongly stimulate plant growth and boost their defense mechanisms. Forest wardens coat seeds with fungi that produce helpful mycorrhiza or bury mushroom stem-butts near roots of host trees to speed up reforestation. Mycorrhizal fungi help plants survive drought. Mycelium processes generate heat, which cuddles the many plant roots when weather turns cold.

Beneath your feet, superhighways of mycelium carry nutrient resources and chemical signals across vast wooded landscapes. This adaptable communal network offers both cooperation and competition between plants and fungi. The system enables trees and shrubs to communicate with each other and share resources. Dying plants dump nutrients into these subterranean pathways, which may be used by growing plants. Tall healthy specimens pump in sugars for shaded saplings that suffer from a lack of light. Older trees act as communication hubs, for they share more links with their neighbors. Chemical signals warn of insect attacks, which prompts plants to increase their output of pest repellents.

The United States Department of Agriculture (USDA) has awakened to sustainable farming. They now recommend methods that benefit fungal networks in soil, as opposed to mechanical tilling that beaks them apart. This resilient renewable approach enables mycelium to absorb more water, use stubble for food and bind soil into air-filled aggregates. Farm suppliers dust crop seeds with mycorrhizal fungi to ensure that beneficial associations start as soon as seeds sprout. This results in higher plant yields, which reduces a need for fertilizers. Fungal antibiotics may prevent infectious organisms from entering plant roots, which diminishes a need for pesticides. Modern horticulture also encourages sustainability. Mycorrhizal fungi are now added to most bagged soil sold in garden centers because fungi seek out nutrients that promote plant growth and increase foliage.

Environmental Triggers that Affect Fungal Growth

Fungi are sensitive to temperature, moisture, chemical signals, gravity, light, ionizing radiation and electric fields. Hyphal tips grow in response to these cues. Mushroom yields also depend on environmental factors.

Fungi need oxygen to grow. Atmospheric oxygen passes directly into fungal cells while carbon dioxide flows out. A build-up of carbon dioxide reduces yields of cultivated mushrooms and in some species causes deformities.

An optimal mix of warm temperature and moisture prompts mushrooms to sprout. A growth spurt always follows heavy rain because fungal cells rapidly suck up water — button cells balloon up, mushrooms shoot out of the ground. Some reach full height in one day. July 2021 was exceedingly soggy in Midcoast Maine and mushrooms continuously popped up all over my yard after downpours. "The best mushroom year ever," said one veteran Maine forager. Mushroom cell walls contain a fibrous substance, chitin, which makes them tough yet flexible. Cell expansion during growth creates such immense force that gangs of shaggy manes and stinkhorn mushrooms are able to bust through asphalt paving. Mushrooms shrivel up and die in low humidity. Growth of a hyphal tube stops when the tip touches a dry surface. Spores with thick walls cope better with drought. Some mushrooms discharge a drop of fluid with each spore to initially protect it from drying out. Mushrooms in temperate zones, such as Maine, contain antifreeze (glycoproteins) to prevent ice crystals from rupturing cells.

Mushroom production drops off in soils with high salinity, though one salt-loving mushroom (*Agaricus bernadii*) has adapted to thrive near ocean coastlines and salt marshes. This species gives off a briny smell.

Most mushrooms grow up towards dim light. Cultivated white buttons are an exception for they fruit in the dark. Brown melanin pigment shields mushrooms from UV rays that damage cell DNA. Melanin also helps mushrooms exploit high levels of harmful ionized radiation for growth. An explosion at a nuclear power plant in 1968 at Chernobyl, Ukraine shook buildings and polluted air for miles around. Technicians who eventually examined the reactor raised their eyebrows and gaped at masses of brown mushrooms on heavily contaminated walls. Analysis determined that the mushrooms had concentrated radiation 500 times above background levels. In addition, matsutake mushrooms were the first living things to grow after the Hiroshima atomic bomb fallout.

Impacts of Pollution and Climate Change

Mushroom formation declines with increasing nitrogen pollution. At least 10% of European species are threatened with extinction due to excessive nitrogen dumping from industry and agriculture. One should avoid picking mushrooms from industrial sites, along roadsides or near mines because they may have stockpiled chemicals or heavy metals to toxic levels. Areas that used herbicides and pesticides (weed-free lawns and old apple orchards) should also be ruled out as foraging locations. The USDA banned some batches of white button mushrooms from China that had high levels of air-borne contaminants such as cadmium. Countries surrounding Ukraine confiscated porcini mushrooms (king boletes) after the Chernobyl nuclear disaster because they contained high concentrations of radioactive metals. Radiocesium was accumulated 10,000 fold by slimy spike-cap mushrooms, another edible bolete.

Climate change has also impacted fungal reproduction, distribution and activity. Europe's mushroom season has doubled in length since 1950. Higher latitudes, such as Maine, are warming faster than other regions. Over the last thirty years, the Gulf of Maine has heated up three times more than the global ocean average. This warming accelerated seawater evaporation which fueled major storms. Over half of Maine's largest rainfall events in the last hundred years occurred after 2005. Mushroom production shifts into high gear when conditions are mild and moist. At the same time, annual precipitation decreased by 20% in certain parts of the state. In these areas mushroom yields declined. A teensy increase in temperature may shift mushroom yields, especially for those that fruit in fall. King boletes (porcini) now fruit later in the year in Maine. Warmth revs up fungal metabolism to decompose wood at a faster rate, which adds more carbon dioxide to the atmosphere and exacerbates the problem. Species adapt to climate change in different ways. A danger is that some organisms may become extinct.

How Fungi Multiply

Mushrooms are fruit bodies that shed masses of spores in order for a fungus to propagate. Spores germinate when they land in an area with plenty of food and moisture; one cell divides to form two identical cells. A hyphal tube emerges from a spore. The hollow thread lengthens from its tip and continues to grow, then branches and fuses to form a new mycelium. Garden shovels help spread fungi because they break hyphae in soil — pieces grow into new individuals. This nonsexual reproduction is simple cell division that makes two carbon copies.

Sexual reproduction is more complex but offers certain advantages. The process shuffles parental genes, which creates individual differences in offspring that may be acted on by natural selection. Increased genetic diversity enables fungi to adapt to environmental change. Occasional mistakes in DNA replication may produce novel enzymes that devour different types of food in new territory.

A mushroom is an organ of sexual reproduction. Fungal sex occurs when an organism has gained enough energy from food. Spores need to be dispersed before a fungus's daily chow runs out. Only members of the same species interbreed. Genetic material (DNA) lies within a nucleus of a cell. Fungal pheromones attract compatible mating strains (A and B) that join to form a new mycelium. At this stage each cell has doubled its amount of DNA because it carries one nucleus from each parent. Branching stops, cell walls thicken and a knot of tubes develops to form a pin stage. Mycelium may have hundreds of pins but only a few sprout into mushrooms. Some have a frayed bracelet-like ring on their stalk, the remains of a partial veil that concealed undeveloped gills of a young button mushroom. A universal veil encloses an entire button of other species. This tears as a mushroom develops to leave flaky scales on a mature cap and a bulbous cup at a foot of its stalk. Scales wash off with rain. All these features are present in fly agaric mushrooms. An orgy of secual bonding takes place in fertile flesh beneath a mushroom cap as nuclei from two parents fuse together. Cell division swiftly follows to produce four daughter cells (spores) each with single copy of DNA. This process rearranges genes from two mating types between four spores. They drift towards tips of club-shaped cells to settle on tiny projections. Flurries of ripe spores drop down.

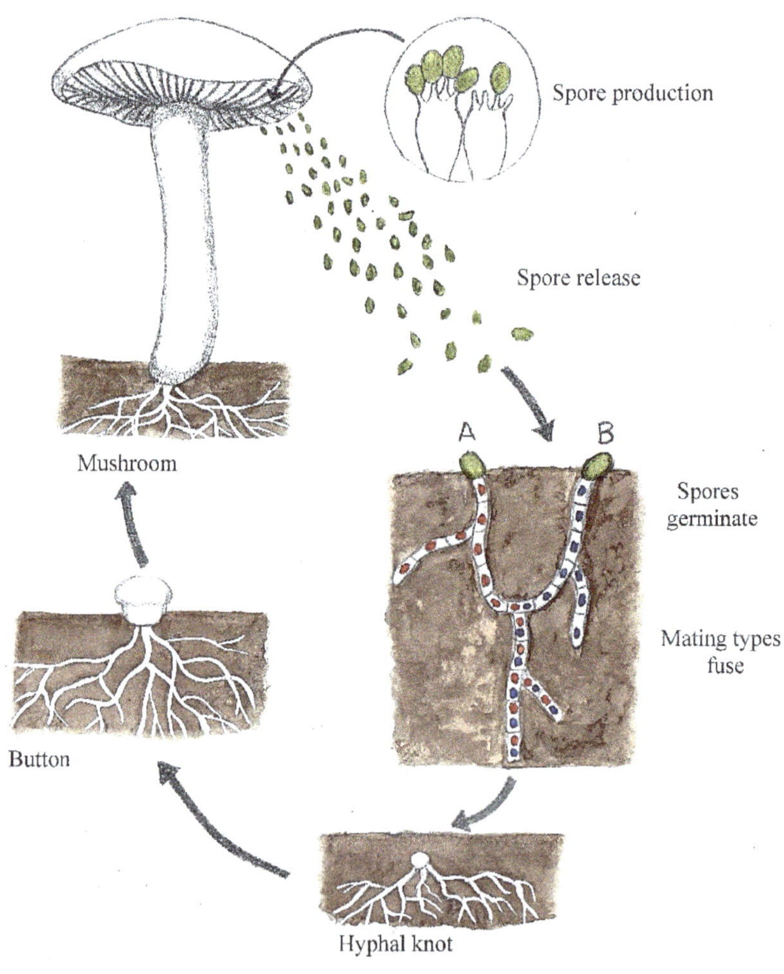

Life cycle of a cap mushroom.

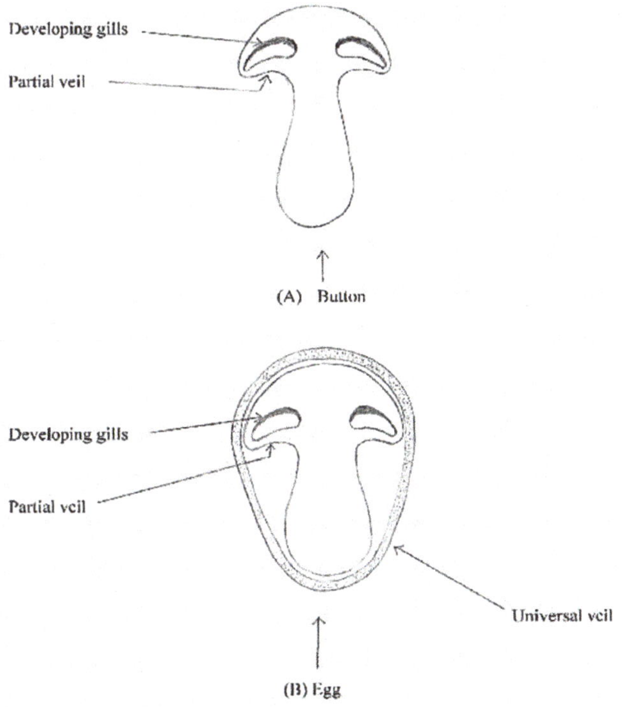

Button and egg stages of gilled mushrooms.

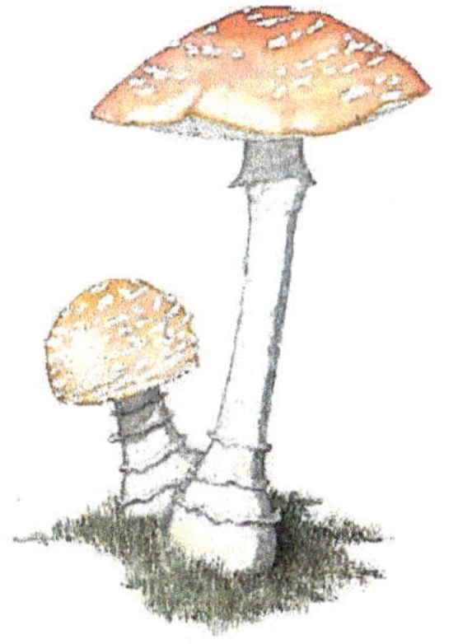

Fly agaric *Amanita muscaria*. Caps of a N. American variant are more yellow/orange than red.

Spores are shed from blade-shaped gills, blunt ridges or spines that increase the amount of surface area for spore production. Other mushrooms have long, narrow, rigid tubes that open on the fleshy underside of a cap. Tiny tube openings resemble pores of human skin or pricks on a silk pincushion. Short-lived mushrooms rapidly disperse spores. Huge numbers are shed to ensure species survival. Estimates for a single mushroom are roughly 30,000 spores per second, billions of spores per day. Spores germinate to form a new mycelium — the life cycle starts all over again.

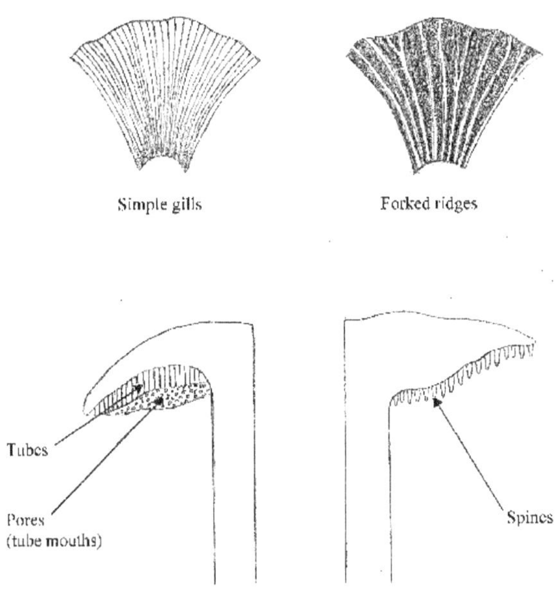

Spore-bearing features of cap mushrooms.

Sexual reproduction in morels differs from that in fruit bodies with gills, spines or pores. Morels produce spores in indentations that give their caps a honeycomb appearance. After hyphae from two different mating types join, they form a hard resting body that can survive drought or high temperature. A morel resting body may hibernate for years, but wakes up when optimal temperature and moisture return to produce a mushroom. Spores huddle in sausage-shaped sacs that lie in shallow pits on the surface of morel caps. Mature spores are violently shot out.

Woodland creatures also play a role in scattering fungal spores, which helps a fungus to multiply in new habitats.

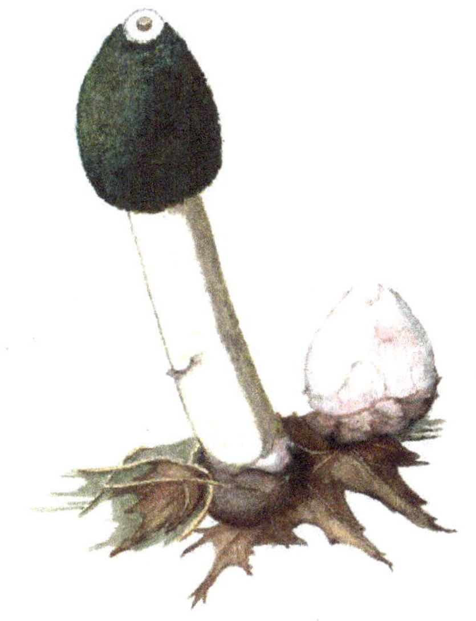

Ravenel's stinkhorn, *Phallus ravenelii.*

Insects fly towards a dung-like stench of phallic-shaped stinkhorns to savor their sweet taste. Legs of insects pick up spores when they clamber over a gooey mass that clings to a stinkhorn's cap. Spores are released when bugs fly about.

Invertebrates nibble on a wide variety of wild mushrooms. Snails and slugs crawl at night towards an eerie, dim, green light that glows from gills of jack-o'-lanterns and mycelium of honey mushrooms. Spores catch a ride on invertebrate bodies and shells.

Prancing deer, lumbering bears and inquisitive squirrels stop to munch on mushrooms. Ingested spores become dispersed when animals drop their feces. A pungent smell from buried truffles lures wildlife that distribute the spores. Truffle mushrooms grow in natural Maine habitats, but the highly prized white species is confined to Europe. Foodies hand over huge amounts of cash for wild white truffles because pigs or specially trained dogs are required to snuffle them out.

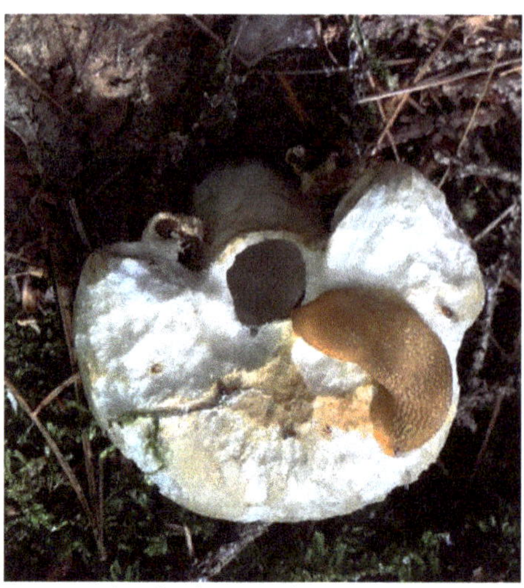

'A Slug's Feast'. Betsy Bass.

How Fungi Defend Their Patch

Mycelium discharges chemical weapons to kill or inhibit growth of microbial invaders that compete for food. The potential of antibiotics was first recognised in 1928 by Scottish physician and microbiologist, Alexander Fleming — a *Penicillium* mold contaminant had halted growth of a bacterial pathogen in a petri dish. The inhibitory fungal substance, named penicillin, was subsequently developed commercially for human use and became available in 1942. Penicillin saved lives of thousands of wounded soldiers in the Second World War. This antibiotic revolutionized medicine, because it stopped certain infectious bacteria in their tracks, yet was nontoxic to human cells. Alexander Fleming shared a Nobel Prize in physiology and medicine with Howard Florey and Ernst Chain for their work on curing bacterial diseases with penicillin. All knelt before the Queen to become knighted in honor of their important scientific breakthrough. Scientists tweaked the chemical structure of penicillin to make broad spectrum ampicillin, carbenicillin and oxacillin without decreasing potency. Fungi produce a huge armory of antibiotics, but only a few land in drugstores as most are toxic to human cells. Therapeutic ones include cephalosporin that targets a broad range of bacteria and griseofulvin, an antifungal agent for ringworm.

Eastern and western cultures approach illness in different ways. Western medicine primarily treats disease with drugs such as penicillin. Chinese healers emphasize prevention with a healthy lifestyle to maintain harmony with nature. They believe that illness reflects imbalance.

Traditional Chinese medicine tries to restore health through natural therapeutic remedies such as mushrooms. Both cultures have adopted fungal cures.

Humans and bacterial pathogens engage in an endless battle — resistant mutants emerge as fast as we develop new antibiotics to destroy them. Bacterial resistance to antibiotics has risen especially in hospitals. Newly discovered mushrooms with unique antibacterial and antiviral compounds may provide a means to combat bacterial-resistant pathogens and new mutant strains of infectious viruses.

Antibiotics of tree polypores (shelf mushrooms with pores instead of gills) might save honeybee colonies from being wiped out by viral infections. In recent years, bee colony losses of 40 – 60% in America had a significant economic fallout because honeybees pollinate about a third of farm crops. Field trials of polypore extracts significantly reduced levels of deformed honeybee wings caused by a virus. Reishi and tinder conk mushrooms reduced viral numbers and extended a honeybee's life. Bees in natural habitats are protected because they sip mycelium droplets that contain complex sugars to fight viruses. Before the 1940s, most farms in the United States had diversified crops and beehives. Modern, mass production, single-crop farming that trucks in bees fed solely on sugar water makes them more vulnerable to disease.

A few fungi produce chemical insecticides. Fly agaric mushrooms acquired their name from medieval times, when peasants floated pieces of a cap in milk to kill flies. Indigenous Americans of the west coast burned an artist's conk to repel insects. A smoldering piece of dried chicken-of-the-woods (a shelf mushroom that grows on trees) drives off mosquitos, a useful tip when camping in Maine. The Environmental Protection Agency (EPA) has encouraged studies of mycelium extracts as biopesticides for termites, carpenter ants and flies, because this approach is less toxic to an ecosystem.

FORAGING MUSHROOMS IN MAINE

Background

From spring through fall, mushrooms thrust their way through grass, soil and leaf litter in Maine's vast expanse of mixed deciduous and coniferous forests. Indigenous Wabanaki have collected mushrooms to round out their family's diet for millennia. Settlers have foraged mushrooms since Maine was part of Massachusetts and gathering food from nature has become increasingly popular in recent years. More enthusiasts scour Maine woods for yummy mushrooms with health benefits.

Fall is a reliable season to find a wide range of species. Mushroom formation is influenced by local weather patterns. They sprout during damp conditions and experienced foragers stay home after a windy spell, which tends to dry up ground.

Maine public lands offer recreational gathering, but this practice is forbidden in state parks. You also need to obtain permission from landowners to forage on their property.

Most Mainers use sustainable harvesting techniques to collect mushrooms. Baskets in hand they tramp through woodlands for that sheer pleasure of gathering free food from nature. Pockets and backpacks are stuffed with field guides, collection bags, notebooks and pens, perhaps a brush to remove dirt, a paring knife or a magnifying lens. Pant legs are stuffed into socks to ward off ticks and most people bring gloves along, as chanterelles often grow near poison ivy.

Toxic Mushrooms

A Cautionary Maine Rhyme

An arrogant fool from Muscongus
Claimed he knew all there was about fungus.
I need no advice,

I eat what looks nice.
So now he's no longer among us.

—Dimitri Stancioff, scientist and
mushroom forager, Camden, Maine.

(Marley 2010).

Some Maine mushrooms are poisonous and a few are deadly even if consumed in tiny quantities. Seasoned mycologists most strongly advise that you learn to identify deadly species in various stages of growth and separate your specimens with notes on their habitat in case you mistakenly pick a poisonous type. Mushrooms with closed caps should be left alone to avoid lethal varieties in a closed egg stage.

BEWARE! NO CHEMICAL TEST NOR CLEAR-CUT RULE DISTINGUISHES EDIBLE FROM TOXIC TYPES.

The genus *Amanita* has a number of poisonous species. Their amatoxins and phallotoxins damage living cells, and cause 80 – 90% of fatal mushroom poisonings worldwide. The most deadly mushrooms are destroying angels and death caps. Ghostly-white fruit bodies of destroying angels appear in September to early October throughout Maine, but thankfully bear little resemblance to edible mushrooms. Severe abdominal cramps, vomiting and diarrhea occur six to twenty-four hours after ingesting a destroying angel. The patient may appear to recover, but then the toxins start to shut down the liver and compromise the kidneys, which may lead to death in four to six days. There is no specific antidote. Silymarin (extracted from milk thistle) may be taken to slow poison absorption. In Europe they push fluids

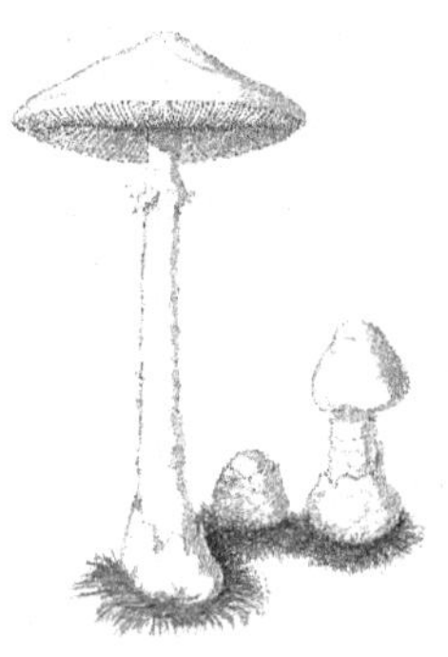

Destroying angel, *Amanita bisporigera* is the most common species in Maine.

into a patient to try and flush out the toxins. American fatalities from this mushroom average two per year. Death caps are the most deadly of all *Amanitas*. Common in Europe, they do grow in parts of New England but so far only one has been reported in Maine. Seasoned mycologists advise newbie foragers to steer clear of little brown mushrooms, a large group that are challenging to identify. Some are mildly poisonous (hallucinogenic), others contain deadly amatoxin.

Gyromytrin, a toxin found in false morels initially causes vomiting and

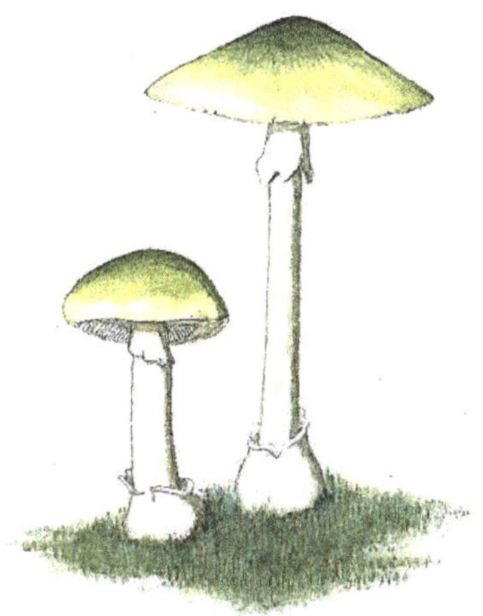

Death cap, *Amanita phalloides.*

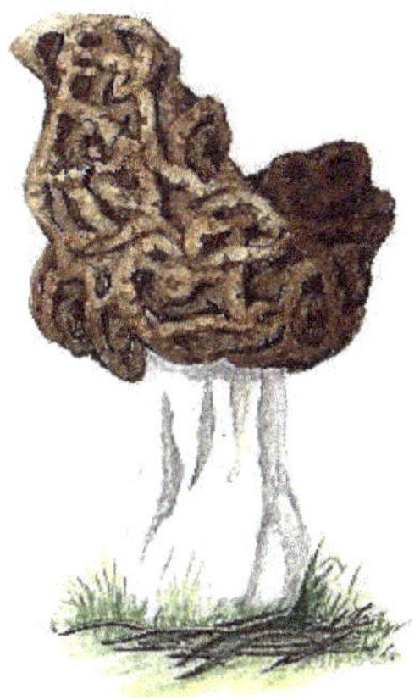

Poisonous false morel, *Gyromitra esculenta*.

diarrhea but subsequently acts on a central nervous system and causes liver damage, which may result in death. The water-soluble vaporous poison has a delayed reaction — symptoms occur days after ingestion.

Muscarine is an alkaloid found at highly toxic levels in a diverse group of gilled mushrooms, primarily in the genera *Clitocybe* and *Inocybe* (little brown mushrooms). The acronym, SLUDGE, is used to describe muscarine symptoms — salivation, lacrimation, urination, defecation, gastrointestinal distress and emesis (vomiting). Atropine, a muscle relaxant, has been successfully used as an antidote. Muscarine was first isolated from fly agaric (*Amanita muscaria*), but concentrations in this mushroom are much lower. Though poisonous and psychoactive, fly agaric mushrooms are seldom lethal. Agitation, vomiting and dizziness occur one to three hours after ingestion. These symptoms may be followed by deep sleep. Seizures sometimes result if these mushrooms are eaten in large quantities. The yellow/orange variant of fly agaric is common throughout our state in fall.

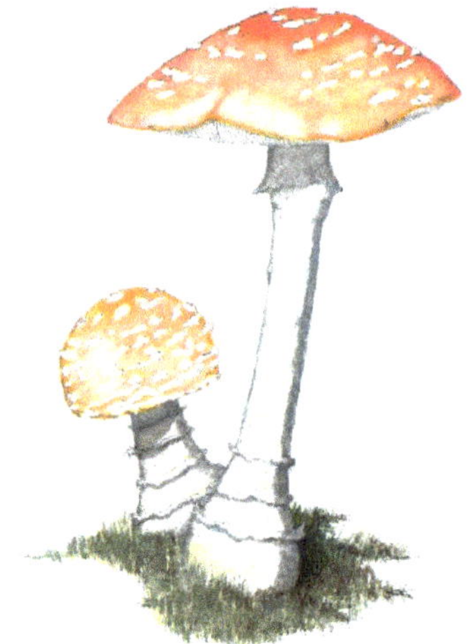

Fly agaric, *Amanita muscaria.*

Wart-covered pigskin puffballs grow in Maine. They are poisonous to some people. Mature specimens have grey to purple-black flesh inside.

Some old field guides, including Audubon's 1981 classic manual, considered lilac-brown boletes edible, yet they cause vomiting and diarrhea in

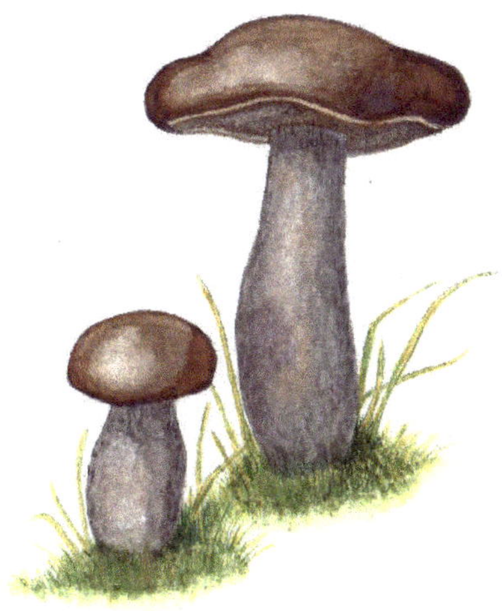

Lilac-brown bolete, *Sutorius (Tylopilus) eximius.*

roughly half of consumers. They are commonly found in forests from August through October. Poisonings from this group have risen in recent years in Maine and these mushrooms should be bypassed. Boletes that have blue markings or stain your hands blue are toxic to most people. Birch boletes, also known as scaber stalks (*Leccinum* species), are often problematic as approximately 3% of all

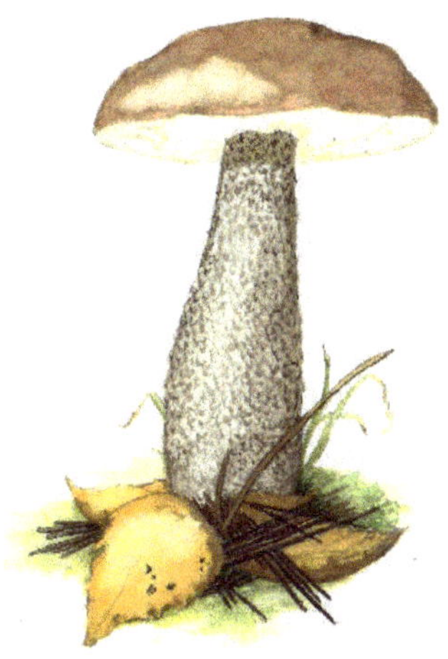

Birch bolete (a scaber stalk), *Leccinum scabrum*.

poisonings are from this group. Over one hundred scaber stalk species grow in North America yet most field guides mention only a few. The boletes in general are notoriously difficult to identify and as interest in foraging has grown over recent years so have mushroom poisonings from this group.

Several varieties of mushrooms contain psychoactive compounds such as psilocybin and related indoles, ibotenic acid and muscimol. Though non-fatal, they can cause dangerous fevers in toddlers and infants.

Your wisest option is to stick with an expert who can distinguish between edible and toxic mushrooms. As one veteran forager said, "You need to be darn sure before you eat 'em."

Most poison cases arise because of misidentification or accidental ingestion by youngsters. Eighty percent of calls to Northern New England Poison Center are from frantic parents of young symptom-free kids found holding a mushroom. The center receives thousands of calls about wild mushrooms (800-222-1222) and will offer advice if you suspect a toxic one. Fewer than 5% of people require hospitalization, under 1% have severe symptoms. Maine mycologist Greg Marley has been one of their consultants for over sixteen years. He noted that an upswing of interest in collecting wild mushrooms over the last six years corresponded to an increase in poisonings with a few serious cases. Further information on poisonous species identification may be obtained from Michaeline Mulvey (North American Mycological Association, 207-737-8695). Antitoxins are available for most cases if you can identify a culprit.

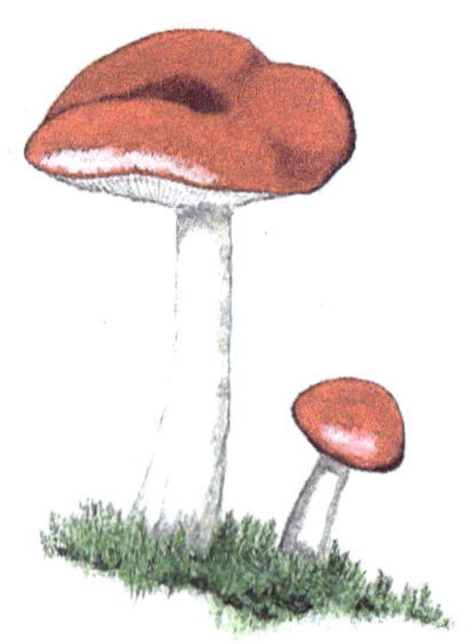

The sickener, *Russula emetica*.

Less is known about mushrooms that cause digestive distress. Gastric problems may arise if too many mushrooms are consumed at one time, or they are eaten over consecutive meals. Blewits, chicken-of-the-woods and morel mushrooms are considered edible, yet are toxic when undercooked

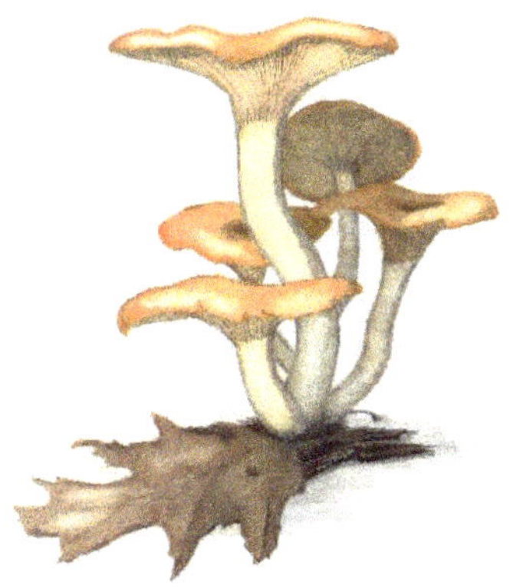

Poisonous jack-o'-lantern (false chanterelle), *Omphalotus illudens*.

or swallowed raw. Their toxins are neutralized by heat. *Russula emetica*, even cooked, makes you vomit within minutes. Hence its nickname, the sickener. Young ones are readily identified by their smooth, flat, sticky red caps, white stalks and brittle white gills. This species often springs up in damp humus near bases of conifers or on mossy bogs. Pumpkin colored jack-o'-lantern mushrooms contain a toxin that gives you severe abdominal cramps and diarrhea five to seven hours after they are ingested. They grow in dense clumps near the base of trees, sometimes more than fifty fruit bodies per cluster.

A common ink cap is a fine edible but contains heat-stable coprine that quickly reacts with alcohol in wine, beer or cocktails to cause flushing, nausea, vomiting or heart palpitations. Symptoms decrease in eight to forty-eight hours, though they return if you drink booze up to seventy-two hours after ingesting an ink cap. This mushroom, also known as tippler's bane, was used to treat chronic alcoholism before pharmaceutical drugs came on the market.

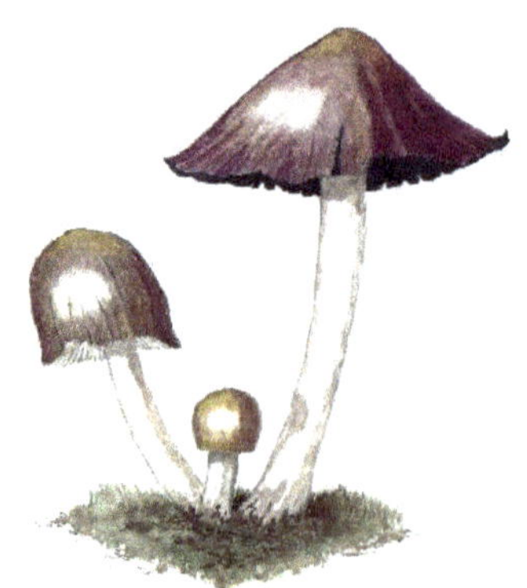

Common ink cap, *Coprinopsis atramentaria*.

Individuals react differently to consuming certain wild mushrooms — some people are allergic. Fungal cell walls contain compounds that may cause indigestion, or gastric issues arise from a type of wood a mushroom used for growth.

You may find Greg Marley pointing out features of different wild mushrooms to enthusiasts on woodland treks or at his lectures throughout Maine. Greg's passion for mushrooms began fifty years ago, when he moved from New Mexico to Maine. He sent out a survey in 2007 to people who had attended his mushroom courses and followed up with a more extensive questionnaire in winter of 2019 to 2020. Greg received 245 responses, close to 200 lived in Maine. Eighty-five percent of participants reported they had never been sick from eating wild mushrooms. Those that did fall ill claimed false identification, or symptoms appeared only after consuming a large quantity at one sitting. A couple of survey participants tolerated maitake, morels and shaggy manes well at first, but developed gastric issues after wolfing them down for days. Although a large clump of maitake may weigh up to twenty pounds, one must avoid a temptation to tuck into this mushroom over several consecutive meals. Even black trumpets cause diarrhea if you eat too many over three days. The most common intolerance was with chicken-of-the-woods and honey mushrooms. Raw or undercooked, everyone becomes sick from these varieties. Some people are unable to tolerate even well-cooked ones. They may be fine if picked off hardwoods, but you might become sick from specimens collected off white pine or spruce. Other survey respondents had gastric issues after eating hedgehog or lobster mushrooms.

Prudent mushroom foragers learn to identify poisonous varieties, always fully cook wild specimens to remove heat-sensitive toxins and eat only a small portion their first time, one that fits in the palm of their hand. Newbie collectors should stick with foolproof varieties that have no toxic lookalikes such as black trumpets, maitake, shaggy manes, hedgehog mushrooms, giant puffballs, chicken-of-the-woods and lion's mane.

Mushroom Identification

This is a life-long process.

Several of Greg Marley's survey questions covered identifying wild mushrooms. Most people employed a combination of resources to help distinguish them, almost all thumbed through field guides, and use of online sites jumped after 2007. Greg is a fan of mushroomexpert.com and mycoquebec.org (in French). Approximately two thirds of survey respondents had attended guided walks or workshops. Over half depended on a mentor for help with identification, either a family member or someone knowledgeable whom they trust.

Most foragers stick to a few edible mushroom species they are sure of or return each year to the same spot to pick their favorites. It also helps to bone up on trees, because some fungi associate with only certain types of wood. Reliable descriptions about mushroom species were difficult to find before 1981 when National Audubon came out with their field guide to North American mushrooms. It is important to note that manuals are unreliable because mushroom shape, size and color may change with age. Spore color helps confirm identity. If you leave a cap (gill- or pore-side down) on glass it sheds spores that leave a print. You can view color by sliding contrast paper underneath the glass, or place white paper under half a cap and black paper under the other.

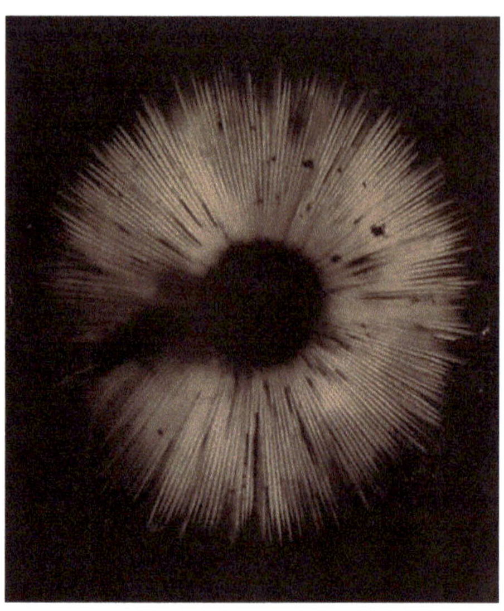

White spore print. Hilary Bartlett.

One may gain experience in identifying edible mushrooms by joining guided walks conducted by Maine land trusts, clubs and select hotels, or by making friends with an experienced forager in the area. Maine Mycological Association holds dozens of forays across the state during mushroom season, mainly on weekends. They have a lending library and offer lectures during winter. Membership is only ten dollars per year, twelve for a couple. David Porter edits their newsletter, *Mainely Mushrooms*. He has led collecting sprees and given talks across the state, including classes at College of the Atlantic and Eagle Hill Institute. Mushroom veteran, Richard Tory, leads an annual fall forage trek in Waterville (put on by Kennebec Messalonskee Trails). This event attracts participants from other towns. North Spore (a mushroom spawn producer) offers a fall foraging class and a workshop on mushroom identification each year at Pineland Farms in New Gloucester, Cumberland County, Maine.

Frank Giglio forages mushrooms in Midcoast Maine. He is a vigorous advocate of local sustainable food and was a featured chef in a *New York Times* bestselling cookbook. Frank first became intrigued by medicinal varieties that grow on trees, in particular chaga and reishi. As his interest grew, he foraged edible ones. The first wild mushroom he ever tasted was a chanterelle and he still loves them.

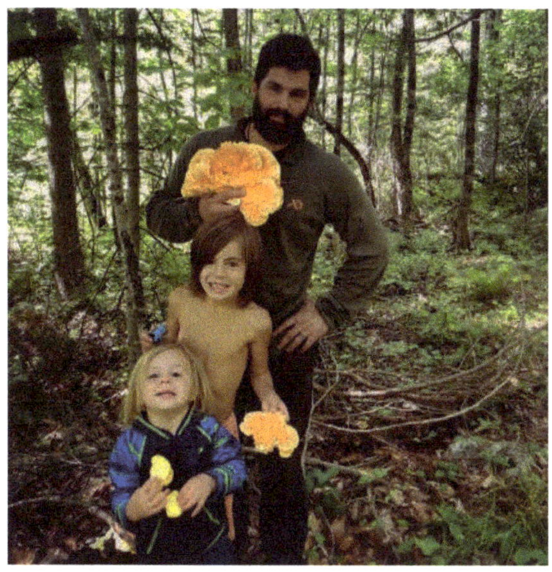

Chicken-of-the-woods. (Courtesy of Frank Giglio.)

Frank also collects ones he is sure of such as chicken-of-the-woods, oysters, black trumpets and hens. Maitake (hen-of-the-woods) is one of his favorites because he loves their meaty texture. Reminiscing about his former twenty-six acre homestead in Thorndike, Maine, Frank noted that oyster mushrooms were most prolific, but he had three trees that produced chicken-of-the-woods. One year he and his kids hit a forager's jackpot — lots of chicken-of-the-woods on a massive old beech at a southwest corner of his lot. "I love it when I'm able to eat a fresh bunch," Frank said. "Then I always dehydrate as much as I can so I can use it in winter." Frank used to produce and sell maple syrup online. He reserved a batch to make a medicinal brand by adding chaga, reishi and turkey tail with a few black currants thrown in. His chicken soup with reishi, turkey tail and chaga functions as a pick-me-up when members of his family are sick.

David Ross, the owner of 50 Local (a bistro in Kennebunk) picks various wild mushrooms for the restaurant. His executive chef uses them as a filling in gnocchi, tosses them with udon noodles and includes them in chicken entrées.

Another enthusiastic mushroom forager is Michael Salmon, an award-winning chef who owns the Hartstone Inn at Camden. King boletes (porcini) are a popular delicacy at his Victorian B & B. His menu also includes a wild mushroom ravioli appetizer.

The Covid-19 contagion sparked renewed interest in finding edible mushrooms according to three of Maine's foraging experts — Greg Marley, David Spahr and Sam Richman. Greg reported that membership of Maine Mushroom Association has doubled since the start of the pandemic. Sam serves wild mushrooms at his Rockland restaurant, Sammy's Deluxe. As cases surged during the onset of the pandemic the dining room closed, but his takeout menu included a marinated, hand-battered, chicken-of-the-woods sandwich. David guides mushroom forays and also loves to cook. He avoids mixing wild varieties with store-bought white buttons, crimini or portabellas (*Agaricus bisporus*) because the subtle flavor of wild chanterelles is easily lost when you mix them with commonly available *Agaricus*.

Edible Varieties

Maine offers a wide variety of edible species. Detailed descriptions of popular ones are described here.

Black trumpets (horn of plenty)

These mushrooms poke up in July through October in Maine near oak, beech or hemlock. Clumps of black trumpets grow in damp areas. Fragile fruit bodies range from one to four inches high. Their dark color makes them difficult to spot, but they make an excellent choice for novice foragers because poisonous look-alikes are nonexistent. Black trumpets emit a stronger aroma than most wild mushrooms — connoisseurs can sniff out a large stand from yards away. Some collectors even claim they smell of chocolate. Hollow stalks support thin wavy-edged caps that roll up and fan out.

Their gills release pink or white spores. You need to carefully clean them with a pastry brush because dirt collects in their trumpets.

Black trumpets were a poor man's meat in Europe. French and Italians call them trumpets of death, yet their flavor sizzles with life. Fresh ones need to be sautéed gently to preserve their delicate structure and slightly sweet, smoky tang. These tasty morsels beautifully accent dishes and also make a great pizza topping. Black trumpets are easily preserved by drying. They may be reconstituted in warm water for thirty minutes, or soaked in a mild white wine such as Sauvignon Blanc for a few days. The broth may be reserved for cooking.

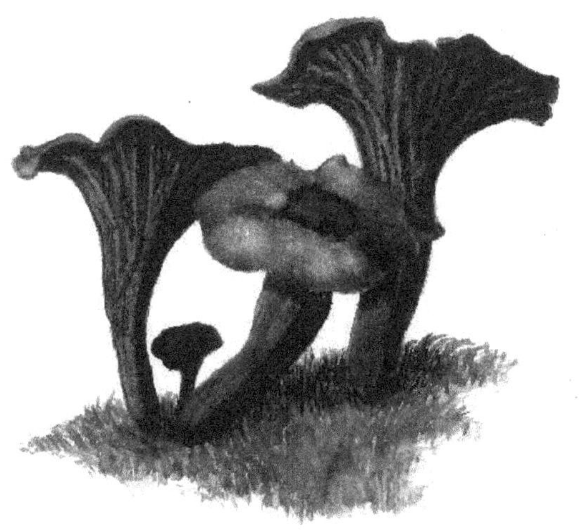

Black trumpet, *Craterellus cornucopioides*.

Golden chanterelles

These common flavorful mushrooms fruit in July through fall in Maine and taste better when first picked. Their glorious golden color stands out on a forest floor, though extensive sunlight bleaches them. Most cap mushrooms live for short periods, but chanterelles may last up to six weeks. Fruit bodies rise singly or in pairs under hardwoods or conifers. Chanterelles prefer warm wet conditions. Caps, convex at first, become funnel-shaped with rolled wavy edges as they mature. They range in size from one to four inches across. Stalks are comparable in length to the width of a cap. Chanterelles have blunted forked ridges that run down their stalks as opposed to true sharp-edged gills. They shed white or pale yellow spores.

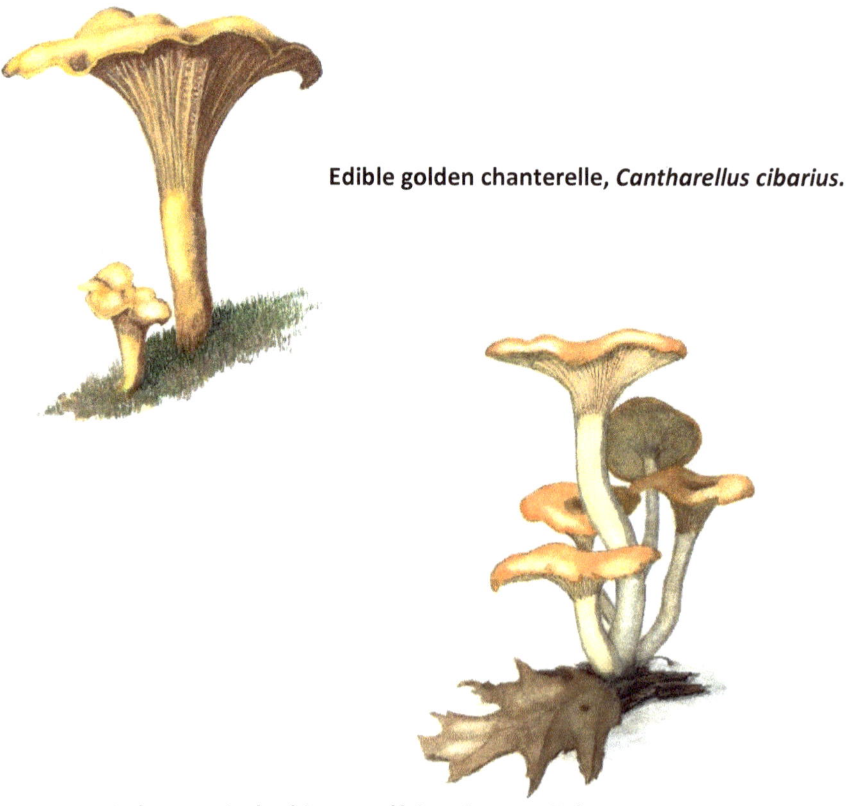

Edible golden chanterelle, *Cantharellus cibarius.*

Poisonous jack-o'-lantern (false chanterelle), *Omphalotus illudens.*

Poisonous jack-o'-lanterns look similar, but their dark orange caps have true, knife-edged, non-forked gills and they grow in dense clumps, often near oaks. Jack-o'-lanterns acquired their name because of their pumpkin color by day and their bioluminescence at night. A cluster of fruit bodies are attached at a central base. If you are unsure of whether you have picked a true or false chanterelle . . . leave it. Jack-o'-lanterns cause gastric symptoms five to seven hours after they are ingested.

Fat-soluble flavors of true chanterelles are readily extracted in simmered butter or cream. Their delicate nutty taste shines in roasted vegetables, soufflés or quiche, but is overpowered by strongly flavored dishes. Some connoisseurs say edible chanterelles have a whiff of apricot. These mushrooms also pair well with chicken or fish.

Morels

Gourmet shops generally carry at least one morel cookbook. Chefs rave over wood morels because of their sweet earthy taste. Their subtle flavor rounds out cream sauces, plus they blend well with omelets or chicken.

Edible morels fruit for one to three weeks in Maine, when wood violets bloom. You may scour woods for miles in spring for morels, yet end up empty-handed. Most pop up in southern coastal regions when daytime temperature reaches 60°F, but occasionally you may luck out and find them further north. Morels may be found near dying elms and woodlands with ash. Hollow fruit bodies grow up to five inches high, flesh is brittle and white inside. White to creamy ochre spores shoot out of shallow pits on their gray-yellow caps. You need to beware of highly poisonous false morels that appear at roughly the same time. As one old saying goes, "If it ain't hollow don't swallow." Convoluted brain-like caps of false ones differ from pitted honeycomb caps of true morels.

Edible morels retain their shape when dried. They must be cooked thoroughly under a long slow heat in order to neutralize their heat-sensitive toxin. You might also want to try a limited quantity your first time, because they produce mild gastric symptoms in some people.

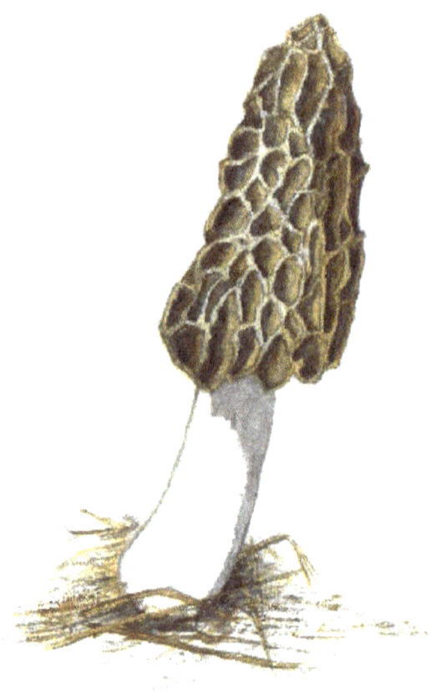

Edible morel, ***Morchella esculenta.***

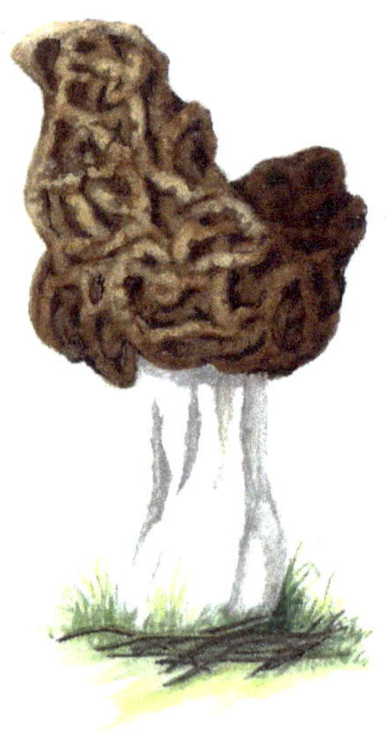

Poisonous false morel, ***Gyromitra esculenta.***

Shaggy manes (shaggy ink caps)

These mushrooms have no toxic look-alikes. Shaggy manes burst forth after the first frost in Maine, often after heavy rain. They may form fairy rings. Fruit bodies generally grow four to six inches high but occasionally reach more than one foot. Caps of young ones hug hollow stalks. Shaggy curls on off-white caps resemble British lawyers' wigs. Bell-shaped older caps flare out. A loose ring (remains of a veil) hangs half way up each stalk. Gills turn from white to black as they mature. Shaggy manes need to be consumed shortly after collection as they rapidly dissolve into puddles of black ink. Young specimens taste delicious when added to stock for risotto or cream sauces.

These mushrooms grow singly or in tight groups in pastures, forests and city wasteland. Foraging should be restricted to unspoiled woodlands, because shaggy manes efficiently concentrate toxic heavy metals from urban sites.

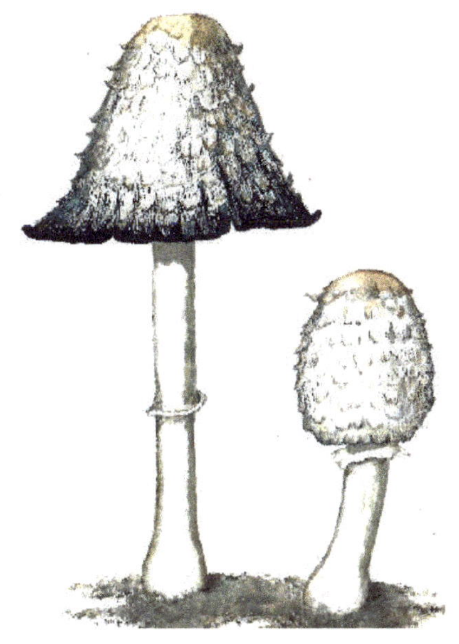

Shaggy mane, *Coprinus comatus*

Hedgehog mushrooms (sweet tooth)

This foolproof variety builds confidence for novice foragers. Distinctive spines beneath their caps are a tell-tale sign, plus they give off a fruity aroma. Hedgehog mushrooms sprout in August through fall in Maine and they may form fairy rings. Short stout stalks support creamy white to pale yellow/brown caps that reach from two to eight inches across. White spores drop down from spines. Young convex caps flatten and become lobed with age. Hedgehog mushrooms are normally intact because insects and slugs avoid them. Fruit bodies turn brittle and crack when they dry out. Hedgehog mushrooms have an ability to freeze in nature yet retain their fresh appearance and flavor when thawed.

Fresh ones impart a sweet nutty flavor with a crunch. They readily absorb liquids which makes them ideal for stocks, or they may be sautéed.

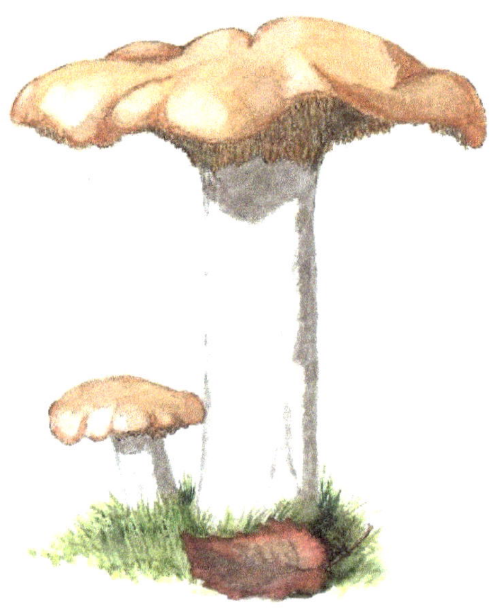

Hedgehog mushroom, *Hydnum repandum*.

Puffballs

These mushrooms are common edibles. Some people refer to them as stomach fungi because they produce spores within an enclosed sac. A splash of rain or a bump by wildlife triggers a cloud of spores to puff out of a surface crack or hole. One immense POOF expels seven trillion spores. Sometimes puffballs explode.

White, fleshy, young puffballs have a mild taste with a texture that is similar to tofu. They may be added to soups or sautéed in butter. Puffballs taste nasty when they turn yellow, tan or green with age. Some newbie foragers start out with a puffball, but try those that are only pure white, dry and solid inside. They should also be larger than your fist in order to avoid eating a lethal, *Amanita*, white egg stage. You also need to beware of poisonous pigskin puffballs with tough-skins that are covered in warts and grey to purple-black flesh.

Giant white puffballs bask in the sun. These foolproof edibles may reach more than two feet across and weigh more than ten pounds. Farmers find them on their pastures, urban dwellers find them on their lawns. They appear from summer to fall in Maine and resemble an abandoned soccer ball at first glance.

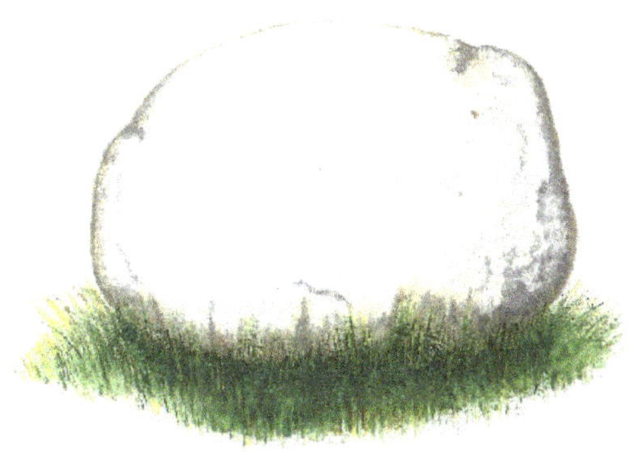

Giant puffball, *Calvatia gigantea*.

Matsutake

Fifteen years ago matsutake were rarely foraged in Maine, but these mushrooms have grown in popularity. They spring up in September through October near pine or eastern hemlock, especially on slopes or near lakes. Matsutake grow up to six inches high. Convex caps sport reddish brown scales, caps flatten as they mature. White gills shed white spores, though flesh stains pinky brown with age. Care must be taken to pull out their deeply embedded stout stalks.

Matsutake's aromatic flavor is brought out when sautéed in nut or seed oil rather than cream or butter. They may also be marinated in soy sauce mixed with oil before grilling. Matsutake blend well in soups and seafood dishes. This mushroom's zesty flavor has been compared to cinnamon or allspice. Many mushroom aficionados rave about their piney resinous tang that comes from coniferous forests where they grow. Others describe matsutake as nasty. Candice Hoydon of Maine's Oyster Creek Mushroom Company claim they "taste like sweaty socks", though she brokers them to a Japanese market. Customers pay an exorbitant price for them in Japan, where they are treasured as ceremonial gifts.

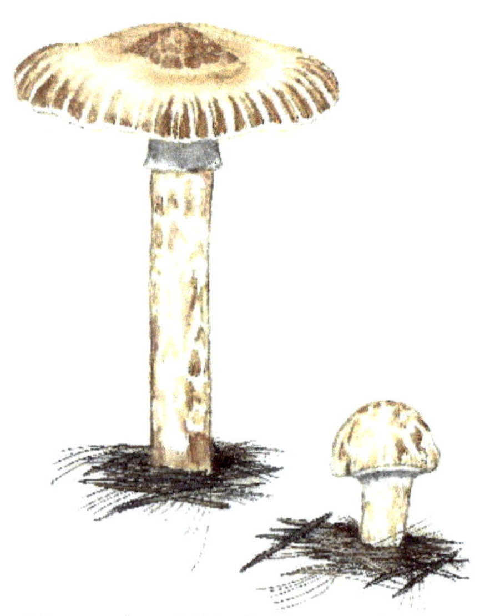

Matsutake, *Tricholoma magnivelare.*

Blewits

Maine wood blewits have bluish lilac to lavender-pink tones. Strongest colors develop in shady locations. They pop up when nights turn cold in fall on composted humus near oaks or other hardwoods, sometimes they form fairy rings. In northern Maine they nudge through pine needles in coniferous forests. Convex caps, from one to five inches across, have inrolled edges. Stalks have a slightly swollen foot. Caps of mature ones flatten and become brownish violet, which makes them difficult to identify. Lavender gills also fade to brown with age. Several lavender and purple mushrooms contain toxins, therefore take extra care when foraging for wood blewits. A spore print helps with identification. Wood blewits shed white or slightly pink spores, whereas those of poisonous ones are dark salmon-colored or brown. If the least doubt throw it out.

Wood blewits have a distinctive spicy taste with a slight bite. They need to be cooked thoroughly, as they may be mildly toxic when eaten raw. Some people have gastric distress with cooked blewits, therefore try only a few your first time.

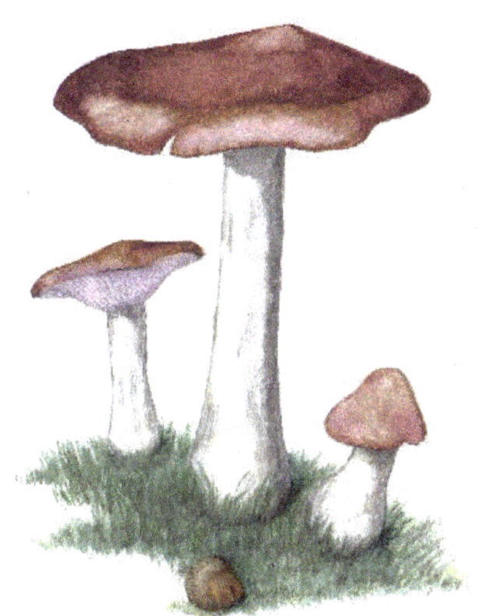

Wood blewit, *Clitocybe nuda.*

King boletes

These muffin-topped majestic marvels acquired the name, king of wild mushrooms, because of their delightful aroma and robust savory taste. This popular fleshy variety is known as porcini in Italy or cèpe in France. They grow under oaks, hemlocks and other conifers. King boletes appear after heavy rains in late August through fall in Maine. Dark veining often cloaks their stout beige/brown stalks as fine as netting on a widow's veil. Young ones have cream or white stalks. Smooth spongy caps grow from two to ten inches wide. They vary in color from a light tan with touches of apricot to a rich honey or a burnt-toffee brown. Caps often become sticky in damp weather. Olive-brown spores drop down from closely spaced tubes that lie beneath each cap. Spore-bearing flesh, white at first, turns yellow to green/brown as fruit bodies ripen. They often become infested with insects or slugs.

Maine mycologist Greg Marley advises less-experienced foragers to be cautious and avoid the *Boletus* group because edible members are notoriously difficult to identify. Field guides exclude some varieties, plus they have a number of toxic look-alikes.

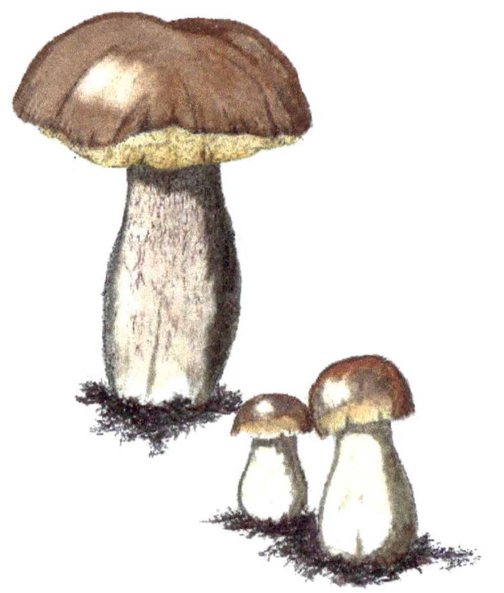

King bolete, *Boletus edulis.*

King boletes have a nutty taste with a slight crunch when sautéed. They hold up in stews, coq au vin and pasta sauces that are simmered a long time. Fruit bodies have a brief shelf life. Drying preserves them and intensifies their taste. Powders made from king boletes impart a strong flavor to soups, sauces and home-made pasta dough.

Other edibles

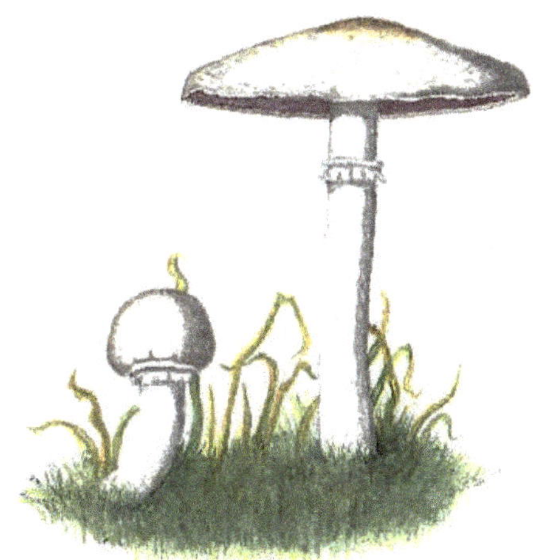

Horse mushroom, *Agaricus arvensis*.

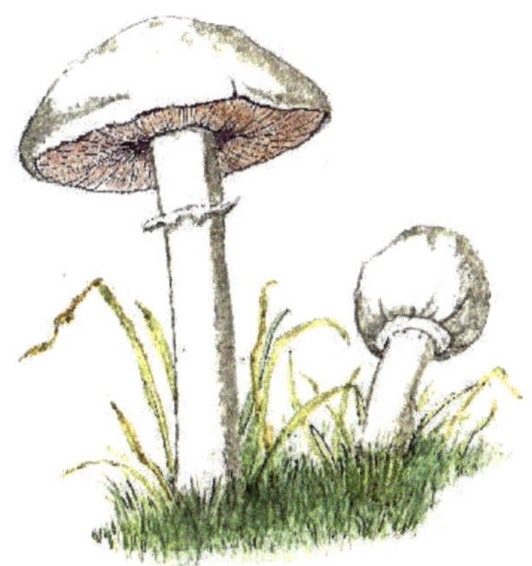

Meadow mushroom, *Agaricus campestris*.

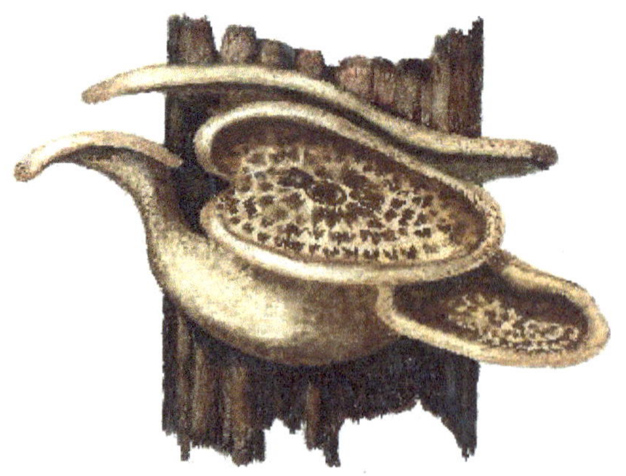

Dryad's saddle, *Cerioporus (Polyporus) squamosus.*

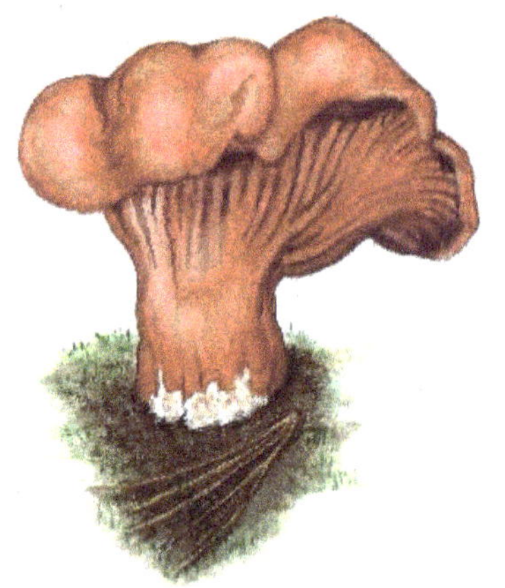

Lobster mushroom, *Hypomyces lactiflourum.*

Horse and meadow mushrooms are relatives of white buttons sold in stores. Some foragers collect Dryad's saddle (pheasant's back), a brown-scaled shelf polypore with overlapping caps, yet it receives mixed reviews as an edible especially if you consume an older specimen. People have eaten lobster mushrooms for hundreds of years. They have a whiff of seafood but their flavor is highly variable, plus older ones are smelly. A red parasitic mold colonizes outer layers of these white mushrooms to give them their distinctive color.

Edible and Medicinal Ones

Maitake (hen-of-the-woods, sheep's head)

Their soft, overlapping, dirty-white, spoon-shaped caps are tinged with brown or gray, which makes them difficult to spot but easy to identify because they resemble a broody hen on the ground. Flattened caps grow up from a central base; underneath, their white stalk structure resembles a cauliflower. White spores drop from miniscule pores that lie beneath each cap.

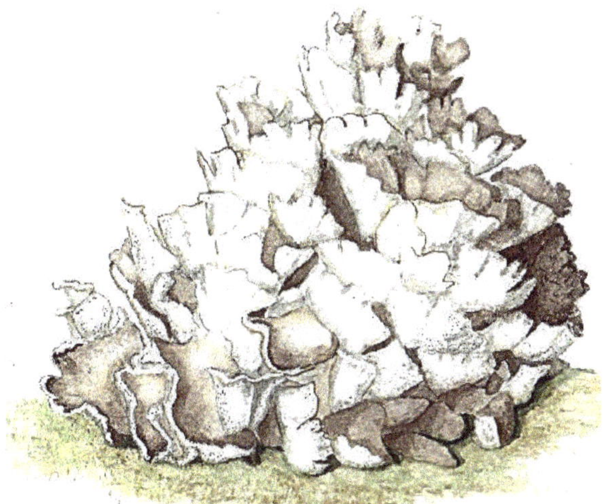

Maitake, *Grifola frondosa*.

Wavy layers of this polypore remind one of ruffled skirts worn by flamenco dancers.

This choice Maine edible has healing powers and no toxic look-alikes. Clusters of fruit bodies appear from late August, after cold nights. Heavy fruiting occurs in September through October in leaf litter under mature oaks and occasionally beech, but rarely other hardwoods. This common fungus is a weak parasite that causes butt rot, though a single tree may produce fruit bodies for decades. They sometimes weigh over twenty pounds and reach up to two feet wide. Smaller fruit bodies make better edibles (before their flesh turns yellow). Fresh maitake provide a distinctive aroma and bold meaty flavor for stir-fries, soups or sauces. Sliced and sautéed in olive oil with a dash of garlic, sea salt, pepper and fresh thyme, this polypore makes a fabulous crostini topping. Italians pickle maitake.

Foraged maitake is rich in vitamin D; concentrations surge if you dry slices in the sun. Hot water pulls out glucan polysaccharides that calm immune systems when overstimulated or ramp them up to fight disease. Preclinical studies suggested that immune regulation by maitake intensified the power of chemotherapy and reduced side effects. Maitake polysaccharides suppressed tumor growth in mice. Other lab studies determined that extracts of maitake killed certain human cancer cell lines. One maitake fraction inhibited replication of several viruses, including HIV-I and hepatitis B. Maitake extracts stabilized blood pressure, lowered cholesterol and regulated blood glucose levels of rodents.

Lion's mane

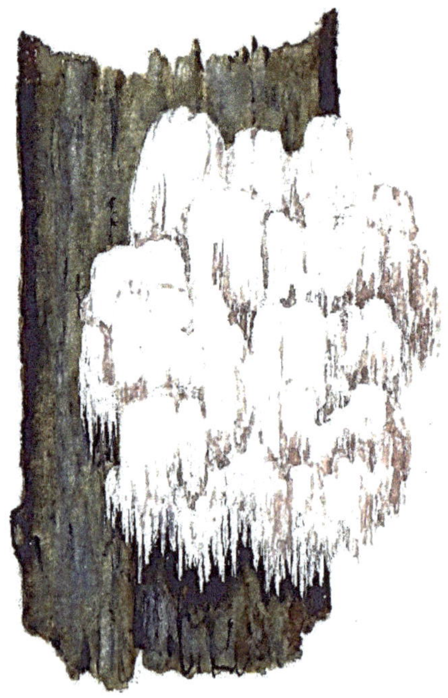

Lion's mane, *Hericium americanum*.

Mature fruit bodies, six to twelve inches wide, branch from a central point into a compact form that resembles a shaggy lion's mane or a mass of snowy needle-like teeth. White or pale yellow spores drop from spines. Long ones resemble fragile icicles, overripe ones turn yellow or brown. The nomenclature of *Hericium* species has changed in recent years. Two types commonly grow in September through October on deciduous trees in Maine, but there are no poisonous look-alikes. Fully-developed *H. americanum* (bear's head tooth) has a branched cascading form with long spines, whereas *H. coralloides* (comb tooth) has more blunt coral-like branches with short spines.

Most medical research has been conducted on *Hericium erinaceus*, which grows in a single clump. Its glucan polysaccharides stimulate an immune response to ward off disease and enhance resistance to mutagens that damage cells. Lab studies demonstrated that extracts of *H. erinaceus* inhibited growth of some bacterial pathogens, lowered blood glucose levels of diabetic mice and passed a blood/brain barrier of rodents to stimulate nerve growth. A small, double-blind, clinical trial in Japan determined that lion's mane (*H. erinaceus*) improved cognitive function in patients with comprehension and reasoning issues. This mushroom is considered as brain food in Asia. Word is out in this country too; baby-boomers have taken note. Lion's mane might prevent or cure patients with dementia and Alzheimer's disease, though large clinical trials have yet to be conducted in the United States. Polysaccharides of lion's mane exhibited anti-tumor effects in mice. Practitioners of traditional Chinese medicine recommend this mushroom for cancer prevention of a gastrointestinal tract and stomach ailments.

Foraged lion's mane should be consumed when white and firm because it wilts when stored. Young white ones turn a crisp golden brown when sautéed. People claim they taste of seafood when tossed in butter. Their texture resembles crabmeat.

Teas made from lion's mane contain beneficial glucan polysaccharides. An alcohol extraction pulls out compounds that promote cognitive function.

Oyster Mushrooms

Their common name reflects the pearly-white shell-like appearance of some varieties rather than their taste. These mushrooms aggressively attack hardwoods. Three species grow prolifically in Maine. One, *Pleurotus ostreatus*, fruits from fall to early winter in over-lapping shelves high up on trunks of mature sugar maples or elms. Their fruit bodies withstand frost. In late spring to early summer, *P. populinus* appears on aspens. A third species, *P. pulmonarius*, fruits on maple, beech and other hardwoods in summer. You should avoid white angel wings on dead or fallen conifers because this variety may be toxic to some people. Their flesh is much thinner and more fragile than oyster mushrooms. Floppy fan-shaped caps of true oyster mushrooms grow up to ten inches wide, one and a half inches thick. They flush in delicate hues of pearl to light gray, cream and blush, though others have brown caps often with a tinge of violet. Gill color varies from white to light gray and yellows with age. They shed spores of whitish-gray or lavender-lilac.

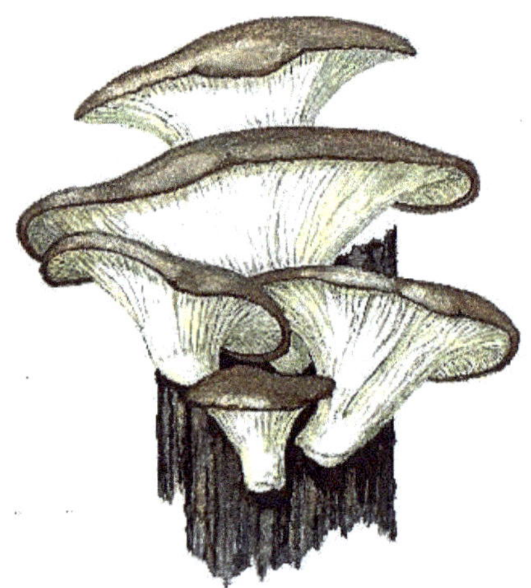

Edible oyster mushroom, *Pleurotus ostreatus*.

Wild ones taste superb in fall. Stalks, if present, need to be removed before cooking. Freshly picked specimens give off an anise-almond smell. Slow sautéing on a low heat is advisable, as their flesh is thick and dense.

Color fades as they cook. They impart a mild sweet flavor and are delicious in omelets or gratins and as a pizza topping.

Drying concentrates the therapeutic compounds of oyster mushrooms. They contain benzaldehyde, an antibacterial, anti-inflammatory agent. Most medical research has been conducted on *Pleurotus ostreatus*. Animal studies demonstrated that their glucan polysaccharides were immune-modulators. One glucan, pleuran, had anti-tumor activity. Oyster mushroom lectins also reduced tumor size in mice. Gills of oyster mushrooms produce a chemical compound that is similar in structure to lovastatin, a Food and Drug Administration (FDA) - approved medicine that reduces cholesterol. Animal experiments determined that oyster mushroom extracts reduced cholesterol levels and regulated lipid metabolism. Extracts of oyster mushrooms also inhibited growth of HIV-I virus.

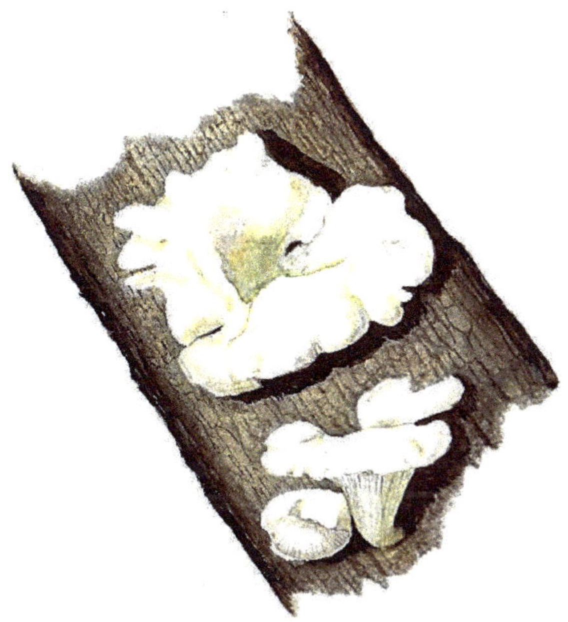

Potentially poisonous angel wings, *Pleurocybella porrigens*.

Chicken-of-the-woods (sulphur-shelf)

This polypore is toxic if eaten raw. Five to ten percent of people suffer from gastric distress even when they are cooked so one should try only a tiny quantity of white young growth the first time to see how it is tolerated. They should always be cooked thoroughly.

This fan-shaped mushroom acquired its name because its texture and taste are similar to chicken. You may easily spot their sulphur-yellow fruit bodies (tinged with orange) in spring on oaks or other Maine hardwoods. A single shelf grows about two inches a week. It may quadruple in size to become larger than a man's hand and may weigh as much as a block of butter by the time late summer swings into fall. White or pale yellow spores drop down through tubes embedded in cream-colored flesh beneath each cap. If you harvest an edge of a young soft one, the remainder keeps growing.

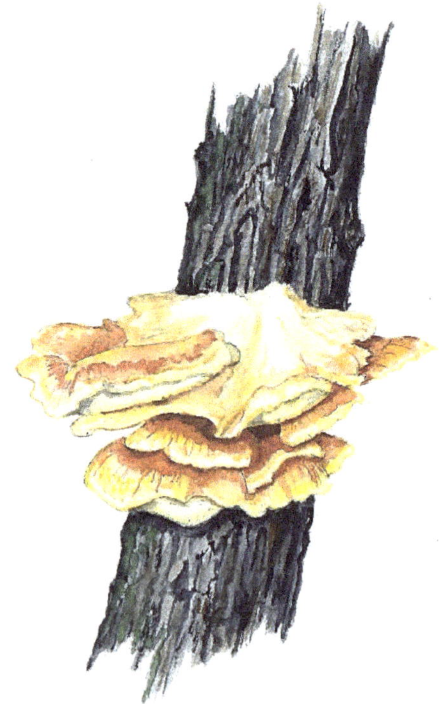

Chicken-of-the-woods, *Laetiporus sulphureus.*

This mushroom blends well in béchamel or Alfredo sauces. Their yellow color is retained when you stir-fry them. They may be preserved by freezing after sautéing.

This tree polypore has a long history of folk medicine in Europe for fighting infectious diseases. Lab studies demonstrated that their antibiotics inhibited MRSA (methicillin-resistant *Staphylococcus aureus*), dental plaque bacteria and pathogenic yeast as well as a human fungal pathogen. Some chemicals in this mushroom helped balance hormones in women with low estrogen levels. Lab experiments determined that chicken-of-the-woods contained anti-inflammatory and anti-cancer compounds. Other fungal substances increased sensitivity to insulin.

———————

Participants in Greg Marley's surveys were asked to name their top ten edibles. Chanterelles and black trumpets won out as the top two in both 2007 and 2020 questionnaires. Below these were maitake, oyster mushrooms and chicken-of-the-woods. Morels rarely made a list because they are difficult to find in Maine but those that did collect them, loved them. Lion's mane, hedgehog mushrooms, various puffballs, matsutake and wild *Agaricus* fell near the bottom of people's inventories. Seasoned foragers with twenty years or more experience placed a bolete near the top. Longtime collectors also included parasol mushrooms as good edibles plus some uncommon ones such as milk(y) caps, which bleed a white milk-like fluid when cut. However, a few milky cap species cause gastric distress.

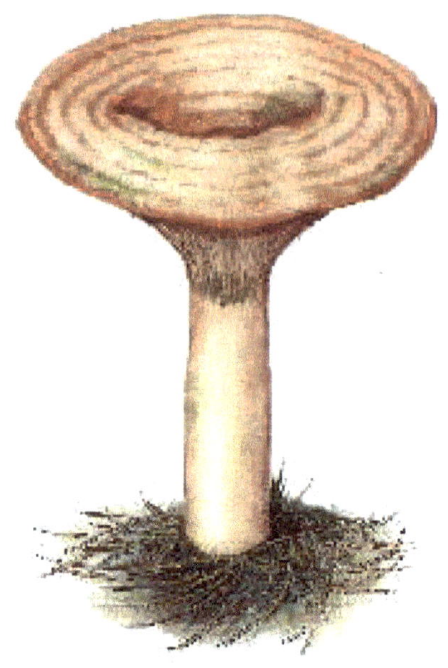

Saffron milk cap, *Lactarius deliciosus.*

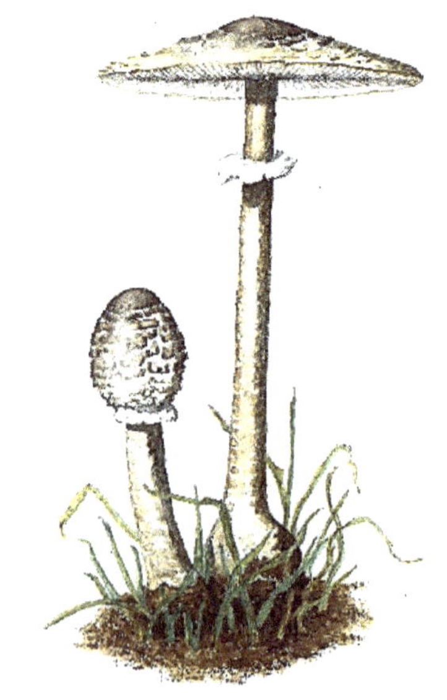

Parasol mushroom, *Macrolepiota procera.*

Medicinal Polypores

Healing mushrooms are commonly encountered in Maine as fan-shaped shelves or hoof-like conks that grow on logs or trees. These polypores drop spores from tiny tubes on an underside of a shelf or conk. A few are annual, others survive up to eighty years.

Hard fruit bodies may be ground into a powder for a medicinal tea. Their full complement of bioactive compounds may be pulled out by a double extraction, alcohol followed by hot water to make a tincture.

Turkey Tail

Concentric rings on fan-like caps come in shades of brown, cream, tan, and gray/blue that resemble the pigments and patterns of turkey tail feathers. This common polypore grows on Maine hardwoods and occasionally conifers. Clusters of their fruit bodies form overlapping tiers on dead or live trees, rotten logs or stumps. Caps grow as wide as your hand; if you touch

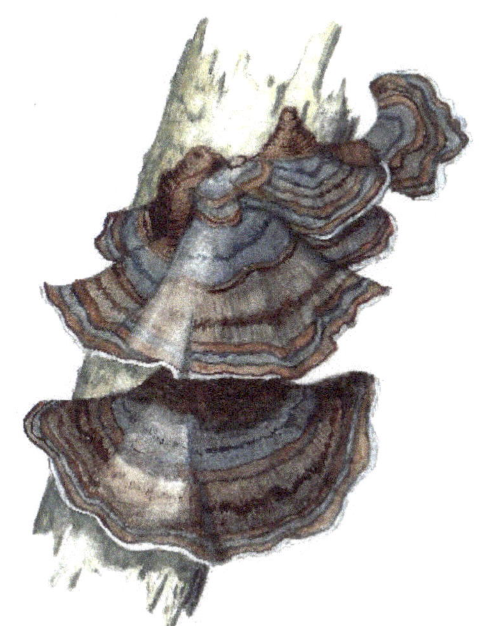

Turkey tail, *Trametes (Coriolus) versicolor.*

one it feels as soft as velvet. A hand-lens is needed to detect their miniscule pores in white flesh beneath each cap. Spores are white to pale yellow. Active growth occurs at white margins from late summer to peak in fall. Old caps are tough and leathery.

Traditional Chinese healers recommend turkey tail for lung disease and liver dysfunction. Healing components may be extracted by steeping strips of turkey tail in water to make a broth or tea. This polypore is one of the most documented medicinal varieties in Asia, Europe and the Americas — primarily used to support immune function. A protein-bound polysaccharide (PSK) and a polysaccharopeptide (PSP) of turkey tail have been successfully used to treat thousands of cancer patients in Asia with few side effects. These mushroom components strengthened immune function of patients who received radiation or chemotherapy, reduced side effects and prolonged survival times. Both PSK and PSP inhibited multiplication of malignant cells and reduced tumor size. A phase I clinical trial, sponsored by America's National Institute of Health (NIH), examined the effects of turkey tail on breast cancer patients who received radiation therapy. Those who received turkey tail demonstrated an increase in cancer-fighting cells of their immune systems. Turkey tail lectins display both anti-tumor and immune-regulating activities. Other bioactive compounds of turkey tail regulate blood glucose levels in diabetics. Consuming turkey tail mushrooms stimulates growth of key intestinal bacteria that help digest food and rebalances an intestinal microbiome.

Reishi (hemlock varnished conk)

You can find a species of reishi (*Ganoderma tsugae*) fruiting from late May to early June in Maine on dead or dying hemlock. Their annual fan-shaped fruit bodies grow up to eighteen inches wide, one and a half inches thick. Stalks are thick or absent. Young red conks look freshly varnished, with yellow and white at a growing edge as well as underneath. Throughout summer, brown spores drop down from tubes embedded in a pore-riddled undersurface.

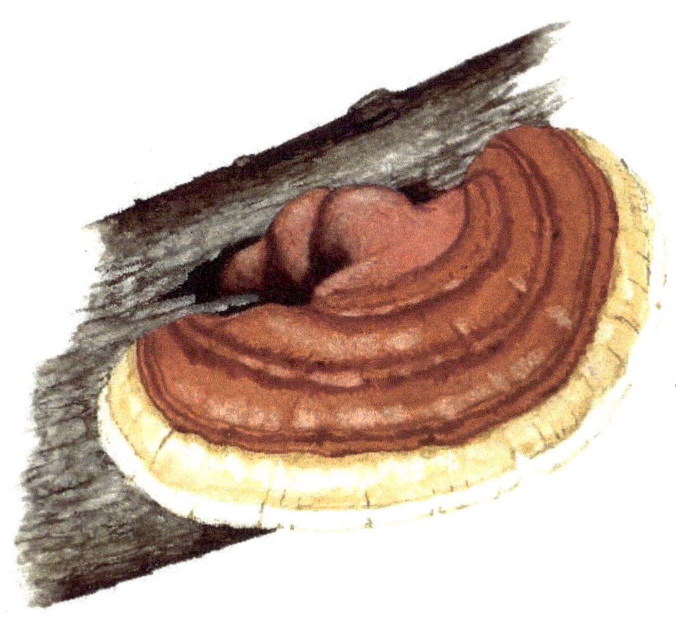

Reishi, *Ganoderma tsugae*.

Most of the medical research on reishi has been conducted on *Ganoderma lucidum* which is native to Asia and Europe. This species is one of the most popular medicinal varieties in China, Japan and Korea, where it has been used for thousands of years to slow down aging and treat liver ailments, inflamed kidneys, intestinal problems and insomnia. In this century, Eastern healers use *Ganoderma lucidum* to treat cancer.

Less is known about the health benefits of the variety of reishi that grows in Maine (*Ganoderma tsugae*), though one study reported that ethanol extracts of this species suppressed growth of prostate-cancer cells. Triterpenes of *G. tsugae* also provided cardio-protection in stress-induced mice.

Because reishi is bitter, it is primarily taken as a double extraction tincture. Immune-modulating polysaccharides are drawn out by hot water; alcohol pulls out oil-based therapeutic terpenes.

Chaga (birch clinker)

This parasitic fungus erupts from wounds of birch trees in cold climates to form a dark, convoluted, sterile mass. Perennial, irregular shaped, black/brown, crusty cankers grow slowly (one centimeter per year) but may reach fifteen inches across and weigh several pounds. Interior layers are golden brown and tough. Chaga primarily flourishes on yellow or paper birch in Maine's cooler mountain regions and near the Canadian border. You need a hatchet, chisel or serrated knife to cut off a chunk or shave some corky chaga from a tree. Brittle pieces rub off. Chaga's fruiting stage often passes unnoticed. A pitted pore surface pushes through cracks in tree bark to release a flurry of light brown spores.

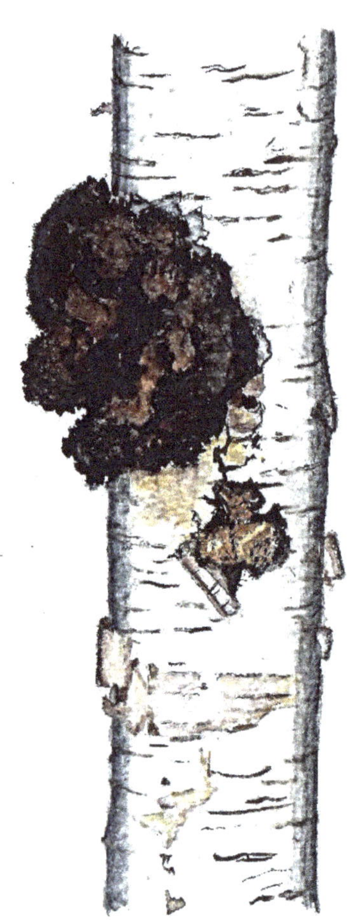

Chaga, *Inonotus obliquus*.

Eastern European peasants have collected chaga from birch trees since the sixteenth century for a tonic to bolster immunity or treat inflammation, intestinal problems and psoriasis. Hot water pulls out medicinal polysaccharides. Chaga tea has been brewed for centuries in Finland and Siberia. Full of tannin antioxidants, chaga's flavor is more similar to black tea than mushroom. Chaga's therapeutic terpenes are removed by alcohol. In the mid-1950s, the Soviet Union licensed an alcohol extract of chaga, Befungin®, to treat diabetes and heart disease as well as breast, cervical and lung cancers. Most people in the west first heard of chaga's healing powers in 1966, when Alexander Solzhenitsyn published his novel *Cancer Ward*. The Russian author believed that chaga cured him of cancer. In recent years, experiments with inotodiol (an anti-inflammatory sterol of chaga) demonstrated anti-tumor effects in mice. Other lab studies determined that chaga extracts contained antimicrobial betulinic acid and regulated blood glucose levels in diabetic rats. A current area of chaga research is pain management.

Sustainable collecting methods for chaga need to be more rigorously applied in Maine because this popular slow-growing medicinal may be in danger from overharvesting.

Artist's conk

These perennial shelf mushrooms acquired their name because artists used them as an etching canvas — the white pore surface turns brown when scratched. These conks thrive in Maine on dead or dying hardwoods such as aspen. Some conks live for decades and reach more than two feet across. You may need a hatchet to remove a hard specimen. Fan-shaped crusty conks have a flat bumpy surface. They produce a new spore layer each year. One conk may release 1.25 million brown spores per hour over five to six months. They float up to settle on top of a conk as a fine dust.

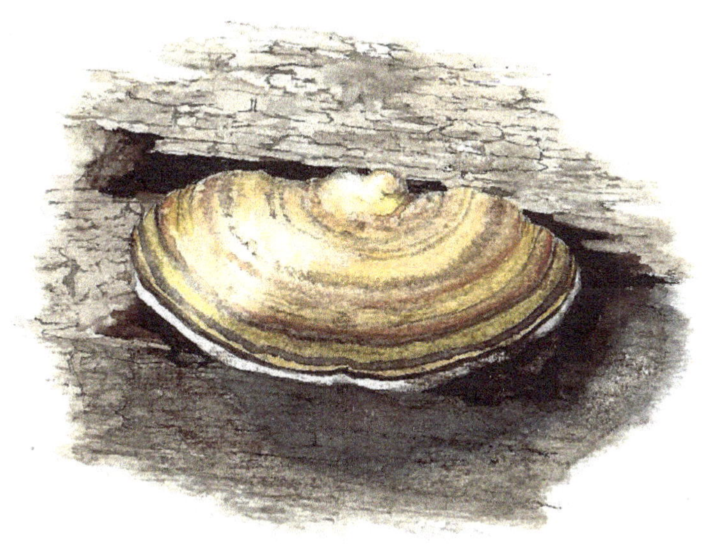

Artist's conk, *Ganoderma applanatum*.

This shelf polypore contains over 400 bioactive compounds. Young, actively growing conks may be ground into a powder to make a health-boosting but bitter tea. A double extraction with alcohol and hot water pulls out therapeutic terpenes as well as medicinal polysaccharides. Studies have been confined to lab experiments. Glucan polysaccharides of artist's conk modulated immune systems to fight disease or reduced inflammation in rodents. These glucans also increased protective mucous secretions in ulcer-induced rats. Extracts of artist's conk regulated blood glucose concentrations in diabetic rats and reduced cholesterol levels. Artist's conk polysaccharides and terpenes acted against tumors. Conks contain antibiotics that combat a range of bacterial pathogens.

I pass an artist's conk on an old sugar maple when I walk down Lobster Cove Road in Boothbay Harbor. Last year I noticed three white/yellow conks developed between March and late August, a possible sign of this tree's impending demise.

Red-belted polypore

This woody perennial polypore grows on living or dead conifers and sometimes dying hardwoods. A shiny red/brown band ends in a narrow cream layer of active growth that starts in late spring in Maine and continues through fall. Older parts of a conk turn dark gray to charcoal. Their bumpy hoof-shaped conks may reach eighteen inches across. White spores drop from pores during wet periods.

Young parts of a conk may be cut off with a knife or hatchet then pulverized. Bioactive glucans are extracted by steeping chunks in hot water to make a broth. Lab experiments demonstrated that these glucans inhibited tumor growth in mice and human cancer cell lines. Conk extracts were traditionally used as a tonic to reduce inflammation of a gastrointestinal tract — recent lab experiments confirmed that acids of red-belted polypore were anti-inflammatory. Tinctures of this mushroom contain alcohol-soluble terpenes that may cleanse a liver and intestines from toxins. Conk extracts reduced blood glucose levels in diabetic rats.

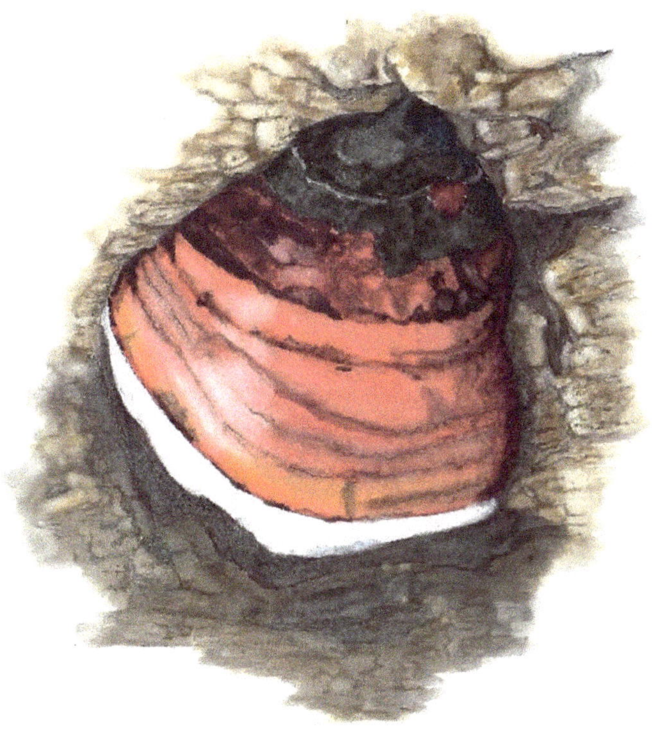

Red-belted polypore, *Fomitopsis pinicola.*

Birch polypore

A 5,300-year-old man (nicknamed Ötzi) found preserved in glacial Alpine ice had chunks of dried birch polypore among his possessions.

Creamy-white conks, two to five inches wide, commonly grow on white or gray birch in Maine. They form annually on trees or downed logs by mid-September in a wet year. Conks turn smoky brown and corky over a season. They curve inwards at their margin; a thickened cap extension attaches them to a tree. An underside pore surface and spores are white.

Our ancestors tore strips from birch polypore for an antiseptic. Present-day lab experiments found that extracts of this mushroom had broad-spectrum antibiotic activity against pathogenic bacteria, viruses and intestinal parasites. Research studies demonstrated that birch polypore glucans and betulinic acid had anti-tumor activity in mice. Betulinic acid also inhibited growth of human melanoma cell cultures. Conks contain a high number of alcohol-soluble medicinal terpenes, which makes double extraction tinctures (alcohol followed by hot water) a better option. These terpenes reduce inflammation.

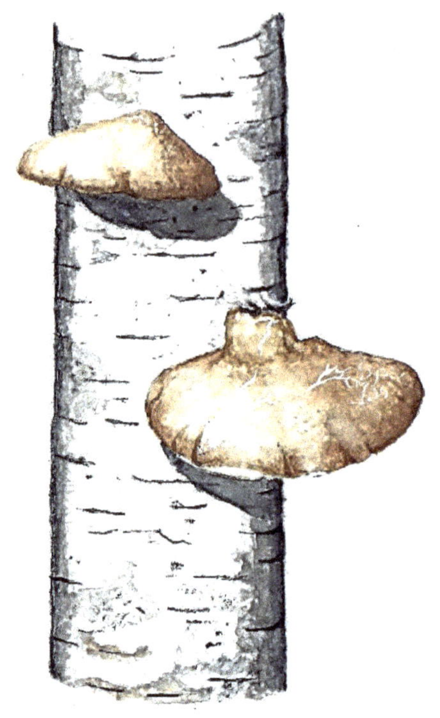

Birch polypore, *Fomitopsis betulina (Piptoporus betulinus).*

Tinder conk (hoof fungus)

Our ancestors harvested tinder conk mushrooms from trees. They hollowed out the inside spongy spore-layer, called amadou, to carry fire. Ötzi (the Neolithic ice man) carried a chunk of amadou in his satchel. In more modern times amadou was used as tinder for flintlock muskets.

Hard, smooth, hoof-shaped tinder conks commonly grow as perennials on deciduous trees in Maine. Silver gray to almost charcoal ones (up to six inches wide) are often camouflaged against bark of trees. Younger, cream,

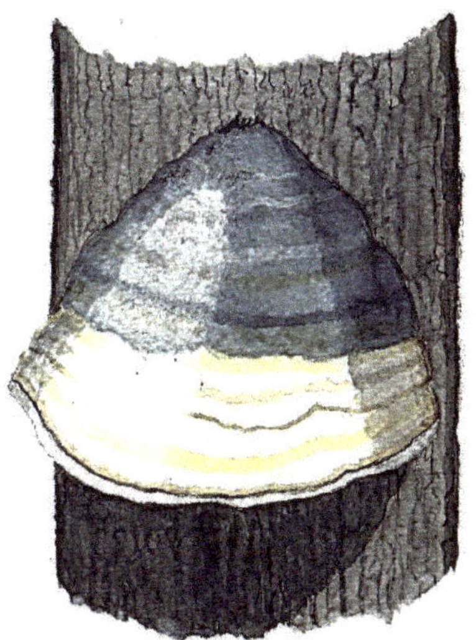

Tinder conk, *Fomes fomentarius.*

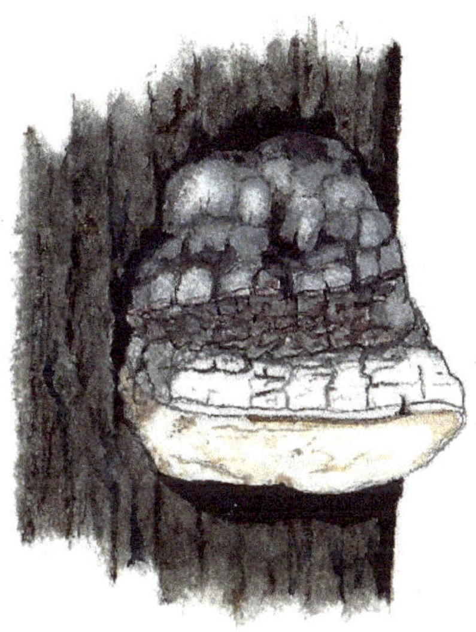

False tinder conk, *Phellinus tremulae.*

growth layers are added after wet periods. Broad growth zones form concentric rings. An underside pore surface turns from creamy white to tan/brown over time. Spores are white.

Since the time of Hippocrates, the inside amadou of tinder conks has been used by different cultures to staunch bleeding and prevent wound infection.

Practitioners of traditional Chinese medicine recommend tinder conk to regulate blood sugar, lower blood pressure and treat various cancers. Although clinical trial data are unavailable, water-soluble polysaccharides of this mushroom exhibited anti-tumor activity in lab animals. Alcohol fractions of tinder conk significantly reduced inflammation in rats. This polypore is regularly used to treat inflamed hemorrhoids in Europe. Laboratory experiments demonstrated that tinder conk extracts inhibited growth of five human bacterial pathogens.

These medicinal conks are harvested during their annual growth period, June through October. A sharp blow with a blunt end of a hatchet removes them from a trunk. The inside spongy amadou may be preserved by drying. Chunks release bioactive polysaccharides after an hour of simmering in hot water.

False tinder conk is a less well-known medicinal polypore. Older conks turn dark gray and crack. Indigenous American tribes boiled them and drank the liquor to treat stomach aches and constipation.

Mushroom Storage, Preparation and Cooking

Freshly picked mushrooms should be cooked as soon as possible to maximize their flavor and prevent spoilage. Specimens may be cleaned with a damp cloth using a downward scraping motion. Ragged skin is peeled away, stalks are trimmed with a knife.

Foraged mushrooms may be slightly dried on a tray before storing in a container or cardboard box covered with a damp paper towel. This maintains sufficient moisture for mushrooms to caramelize when sautéed. Searing also crisps and seals in delicate mushroom flavors but they are easily overwhelmed, therefore avoid cooking wild varieties with heavy spices, too much onion or garlic. Foraged mushrooms are added to dishes that pair with white wine. King boletes (porcini) and maitake are exceptions — their more robust taste blends well with foods that are complemented by a dry red.

Preserving Wild Specimens

Preservation methods enable you to savor mushrooms out of season and support your health year-round.

Drying

Mushrooms need to be dried rapidly to prevent molding. Drying also prevents tiny bugs from consuming freshly foraged specimens. Small mushrooms dehydrate when hung from a string in a well-ventilated kitchen. Larger specimens may be laid on paper towels on a counter. You may also try drying mushrooms on top of a radiator as long as you turn them occasionally, or use a rack in a slightly warm oven (on the lowest setting with the door ajar). Dried ones may be stored in a moisture-proof glass container or plastic bag. You may rehydrate dried mushrooms by soaking in hot water for twenty to thirty minutes; the broth may be used for a stew or a sauce. Dried mushrooms have a much longer shelf life (two to three years) and their flavor increases with age. Throw them in your coffee grinder or pulverize them with a pestle and mortar — mushroom powders add flavor to compound butter, fish, or homemade pasta dough. You may also freeze-dry whole mushrooms.

Duxelles

Wild mushrooms may be preserved as duxelles, a concentrated paste frozen in ice cube trays. Finely chopped mushrooms are sautéed and caramelized in butter with a pinch of nutmeg and salt before freezing. Plop duxelles into your soups and sauces, a quick easy way to add more flavor.

Pickling and preserving in oil

Mushrooms are briefly simmered for five minutes in brine (two parts white wine vinegar to one part water), drained and dried for two hours, then spooned into a sterile jar. Pickled mushrooms need to be mixed with regular olive oil to reduce their sharpness (a strong virgin-pressed oil overwhelms their delicate flavor). You may add a couple of bay leaves, a sprig of rosemary and a few black peppercorns before lids are closed. Pickled mushrooms should be stored for a month before use.

Decoctions

Chunks of chaga, turkey tail and reishi may be simmered for an hour or more to make a health-boosting tea.

Making tinctures

Some medicinal polypore decoctions are bitter, which makes tinctures a better option. They also extract all of a mushroom's therapeutic compounds. Bioactive glucan polysaccharides are readily pulled out by the hot water, but nerve stimulants and oil-based medicinal terpenes require an alcohol extraction. Mushroom tinctures are made with grain alcohol (ethanol) or vodka (100 proof or more) and spring or distilled water. Fractions are blended to yield a product with 75% water to 25% alcohol.

Commercial Mushroom Foraging

Professional foragers supply farmers markets and restaurants with a wide variety of freshly picked mushrooms. Wild chanterelles fetch twenty-four times more per pound compared with store-bought white buttons. Chefs also pay a high price for foraged matsutake. Commercial mushroom foragers guard their secret woodland locations and monitor seasonal weather patterns in order to gather different varieties at their peak.

Oyster Creek Mushroom Company of Damariscotta is a foraging business. Owner Candice Hoydon works with forty professionals who know when and where to look for wild varieties, mainly from information passed down through their families. The Damariscotta Company primarily sells

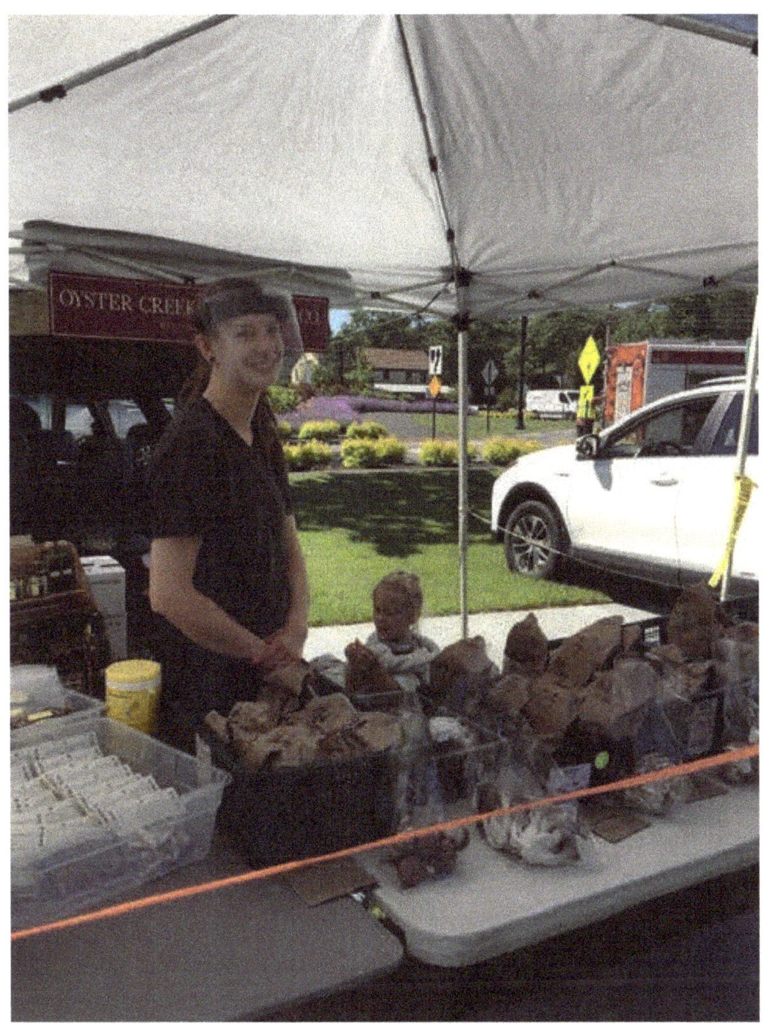

Oyster Creek Mushroom booth at Boothbay Farmers Market (2020). Hilary Bartlett.

to small, New England, wholesale buyers, but one Boston client regularly buys one hundred pounds of fresh mushrooms at a time. I used to buy their freshly foraged mushrooms from Boothbay farmers market. Nowadays, they focus on orders from their website which offers packets of a dried wild mix, a selection of mushroom-flavored oils and mushroom powders, plus a salsa of minced summer truffles in olive oil. Oyster Creek Mushrooms was the first Maine business to offer a medicinal supplement — a full spectrum, fourteen mushroom blend powder designed to improve your pet's health.

White Mountain Mushrooms offer dried edible varieties gathered from forests and mountains of western Maine. They also sell a healing blend. Their range includes chanterelles, black trumpets, matsutake, reishi, maitake, lion's mane, turkey tail, chaga, and birch polypore. You may buy their foraged mushrooms online or at farmers markets in Oxford and Cumberland counties. Merchandise comes in packets or biodegradable cotton teabags.

Some mushroom enthusiasts disapprove of commercial collection. They argue that the fun is in the hunt. Others worry about excessive exploitation, especially of slow-growing chaga.

HEALTH BENEFITS OF MUSHROOMS

Mushrooms are low calorie, low sodium, cholesterol-free foods loaded with beneficial vitamins, antioxidants and minerals, plus many species contain healing compounds.

Nutrition

Our bodies need a regular diet of proteins, carbohydrates, fats and fiber. Carbs provide fuel. Fats keep us warm. Proteins keep our muscles strong and build enzymes, hormones, antibodies and a clotting factor found in blood.

Table 3. Nutritional Value of Raw Mushrooms from Retail Outlets in 12 U.S. Cities.

	White button mushrooms	DV	Oyster mushrooms	DV	Maitake	DV	Enoki	DV
Fat	0.34g	<1%	0.33g	<1%	0.20g	<1%	0.28g	<1%
Carbo-hydrate	3.69g	1%	5.95g	2%	6.81g	2%	8.42g	3%
Beta-glucans	0.21g		0.79g		0.29g		0.62g	
Dietary Fiber	1.45g	6%	2.10g	8%	2.70g	10%	2.80g	11%
Protein	3.00g	6%	2.75g	6%	1.94g	4%	2.66g	5%
Thiamine (B1)	0.05mg	4%	0.17mg	14%	0.15mg	13%	0.22mg	18%
Riboflavin (B2)	0.22mg	17%	0.33mg	25%	0.24mg	18%	0.20mg	15%
Niacin (B3)	2.80mg	18%	5.87mg	37%	6.58mg	41%	7.03mg	44%

Pantothenic acid (B5)	1.36mg 27%	1.30mg 26%	0.27mg 5%	1.35mg 27%
Vitamin B6	0.05mg 3%	0.10mg 6%	0.05mg 3%	0.01mg 6%
Folate (B9)	19µg 5%	6µg 2%	29µg 7%	52ug 13%
Ergosterol*	59.00mg	69.00mg	59.00mg	37.00mg
Calcium	4.00mg <1%	1.00mg <1%	1.00mg <1%	0.40mg <1%
Copper	0.30mg 33%	0.12mg 13%	0.25mg 28%	0.11mg 12%
Iron	0.22mg 1%	0.91mg 5%	0.30mg 2%	1.15mg 6%
Phospho-rus	94.00mg 8%	98.00mg 8%	74.00mg 6%	105.00mg 8%
Magnes-ium	10.00mg 2%	15.00mg 4%	10.00mg 2%	16.00mg 4%
Manganese	0.05mg 2%	0.10mg 4%	0.06mg 3%	0.08mg 3%
Potassium	358.00mg 7%	324.00mg 7%	204.00mg 4%	359.00mg 2%
Sodium	15.00mg <1%	6.00mg <1%	1.00mg <1%	3.00mg <1%
Zinc	0.60mg 5%	0.77mg 7%	0.75mg 6%	0.65mg 6%

Most nutrients were retained at 100% after cooking.
DV=daily value 3/2020. http://www.FDA.gov/NewNutritionFactsLabel.
g = gram (0.0353 ounces), mg = milligram, (10^{-3} gram), µg = microgram, (10^{-6}gram)
*precursor of vitamin D

Haytowitz 2006 (USDA Nutrient Data Lab)

Though mushrooms have numerous health benefits, their protein content is less than 10% of that in meat. Oyster mushrooms had the highest amount, only half of beans, peas and lentils. Protein data, from the USDA, of four mushroom varieties were also in the same low range (Table 3). Note that the data presented here are for wet weight, which is the routine method used by food analysis labs around the world. Reports of high protein content of mushrooms are invariably for data expressed per dry weight and mushrooms have a high water content.

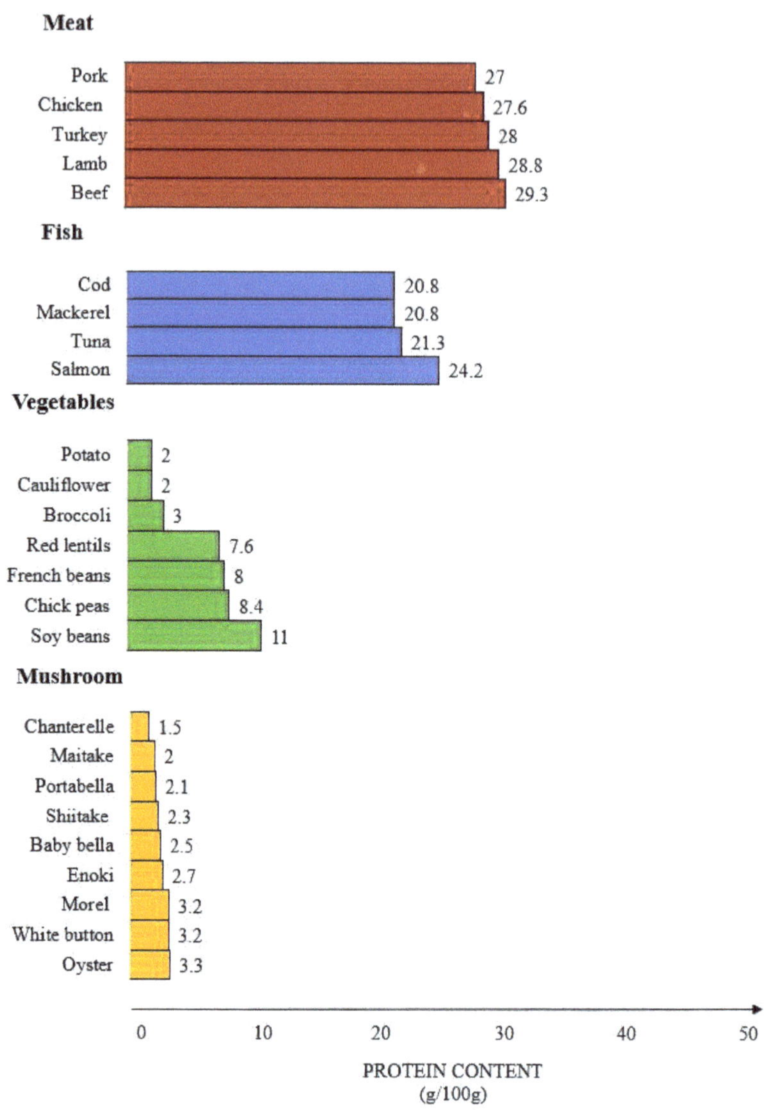

Protein content of various types of food (g/100g). 100 gram=3.53 oz. Gebhardt and Thomas, 2002. British nutrition foundation 2012. Bender 2018.

Mushrooms help maintain a healthy body mass index because they satisfy your appetite without loading up on unhealthy grease and calories. Meat contains saturated fats that elevate blood cholesterol and may cause heart disease, whereas mushrooms contain healthy unsaturated fats. Healthy foods are high in fiber but low in sugar. Several edible mushroom varieties have good fiber to sugar ratios, enoki has the highest score. Chanterelles have the highest fiber content per ounce. Mushrooms are also chock-full of antioxidants, minerals and vitamins that support our health.

Mushrooms contain high levels of ergothioneine and glutathione, two antioxidants that guard human cells from damage associated with Alzheimer's, heart disease and cancer. King boletes (porcini) had the most selenium (an antioxidant) of 126 tested mushroom species. The yellow color of chanterelles is from beta-carotene, a precursor of vitamin A that sidelines as an antioxidant. Many fungi contain brown melanin pigment, another antioxidant. The National Cancer Institute stated that mushroom antioxidants may help prevent some cancers. An extensive statistical analysis by researchers at Penn State found that regular mushroom consumption lowered the risk of cancer. The strongest association was with breast cancer.

The American Heart Association included mushrooms on their list of foods that provide the mineral potassium. Mushrooms have low sodium to potassium ratios, which lowers a risk of hypertension in consumers. Maitake have the lowest score. Shiitake mushrooms are one of the few natural sources of germanium, a mineral that increases resistance to pollutants and disease.

Wild mushrooms are the only organic vegan source of vitamin D, which helps absorb calcium and phosphorus needed for bone growth, and boosts immunity as well as muscle function. Sunlight converts ergosterol in fungal cell walls into vitamin D. Fresh maitake is an excellent source. Three and half ounces (just shy of half a cup) provide 2,000 international units of vitamin D, which meets the FDA's daily value. A similar quantity of freshly-picked wood morels supply 34 – 50% of this recommended amount. Shiitake cultivated outdoors contain five to seven times more vitamin D than those grown inside. Asian countries routinely sun-dry mushrooms to spike levels of vitamin D. Some mushroom growers in the United States use UV-B radiation to increase levels of this vitamin. Mushrooms (except for chanterelles) are a good source of B vitamins such as pantothenic acid (B5) niacin (B3) and riboflavin (B2). Pregnant women often take a folate supplement (B9) to improve fetal health; fresh mushrooms provide a natural alternative.

Americans have started to include more mushrooms in their diet. The United States food service industry is a major financial driver in the current mushroom boom. Their professionals mix chopped mushrooms with ground meat to provide more nutritious sustainable food. The Blended Burger Project started in 2015. Their goal is to mix at least 25% of fresh mushrooms into burgers that are healthier for their customers and the planet.

Healing Mushrooms

Filamentous fungi fabricate fantastic pharmaceuticals. Long-lived polypore conks (woody, shelf or hoof-like fruit bodies) produce an arsenal of chemicals to defend themselves against microbial predators. Some of these compounds cure human maladies. Of 14,000 thousand mushroom species approximately 1,800 have potential therapeutic applications, about 700 have verified medicinal value.

Bioactive compounds are isolated commercially from mushrooms, cultured mycelium or culture broth. Concentrations depend on fungal species, stage of development and growth conditions. Drying concentrates medicinal components of wild mushrooms. Therapeutic compounds may be extracted by hot water to make stocks, soups and teas, or pulled out by alcohol to make tinctures. To date, a total of 126 medicinal functions have been attributed to fungal products. The most important applications of mycotherapy are listed below:

- Kill or prevent growth of microorganisms that cause disease.
- Modulate immune systems to ward off infections, eliminate abnormal cells and reduce inflammation.
- Destroy oxidizing agents that damage cells, which may result in cancer.
- Act against cancer cell multiplication.
- Reduce cholesterol and protect cardiovascular systems.
- Act against toxins and prevent liver damage.
- Regulate blood glucose levels.
- Support nerve cell growth and cognitive function.
- Enhance longevity.
- Maintain hormone balance.

Over the last thirty years, more than a hundred varieties of medicinal mushrooms have been approved for cancer treatment in China and Japan. Turkey tail, reishi, chaga, maitake and shiitake are the most common ones. Potent mushroom chemicals may slow multiplication of cancer cells, regulate tumor genes or increase rates of malignant cell destruction by a patient's defense system. Mushroom bioactive components are used alone or in combination with radiation and chemotherapy to:

- Increase effectiveness of these conventional cancer treatments and improve patients' survival rates.
- Reduce side effects of conventional cancer therapies: nausea, loss of appetite, hair loss, pain, fatigue, and brain fog.
- Protect against bone marrow suppression.

Fungal glucan polysaccharides support our immune systems to maintain health. They ramp them up to fight infections and eliminate abnormal cells, or tune them down to counteract inflammation. Therapeutic glucans break down a few days after harvesting, therefore mushrooms should be eaten soon after collection to optimize their health benefits. Cooking breaks down mushroom structure to release glucans. They survive stomach acid and pass into a small intestine where they latch onto receptors. Mushroom glucans work on functional immune systems and especially benefit people who live active stressful lives. About 650 fungal species from 180 genera produce immune-modulating polysaccharides. Some slow or shrink tumor growth and support cancer remission.

Table 4. Fungal Polysaccharides with Anticancer Effects in Animals.

Mushroom Variety	**Tumor or Cancer Tissue**	**Polysaccharide Origin**
Turkey tail	Lung, breast and digestive organ cancers	Culture medium
Shiitake	Stomach cancer, leukemia	Fruit body
Split-gill mushroom	Cervical cancer	Culture medium
Reishi (*Ganoderma lucidum*)	Anti-tumor	Fruit body & culture medium
Maitake (hen-of-the-woods)	Anti-tumor	Fruit body & culture medium

Fruit body = mushroom
Chang and Miles 2004.

Three fungal polysaccharides have undergone clinical trials in China and Japan where they are extensively used to fight cancer:

(1) Krestin®, a polysaccharide-K (PSK) fraction from turkey tail mycelium, is given to patients who undergo radiation or chemotherapy to boost their immune response and reduce stress on their bodies. Licensed in 1977, PSK is a major cancer drug in Japan.
(2) Lentinan®, a polysaccharide extract from shiitake fruit bodies, is licensed by the Japanese government's pharmaceutical agency to inhibit tumor growth.
(3) Schizophyllan, a polysaccharide produced by mycelium of split-gill mushrooms, acts against tumors and stimulates a patient's immune system.

Some mushroom lectins (glycoproteins) act against cell multiplication in tumor cell lines of leukemia, liver hepatoma and breast cancer, or display immune-regulating activities. Terpenes (hydrocarbons in essential oils) of some polypores kill cancer cells or inhibit their growth. Several mushroom species produce enzyme inhibitors that show potential as adjunct cancer treatments. One fungal enzyme interrupts androgen from forming estrogen, which may limit rapid reproduction of breast cancer cells. Another fungal-derived enzyme inhibits dihydrotestosterone production linked to prostate cancer growth.

Reports of mushroom lab studies and human clinical trials from Pacific Asia, Europe and North America have increased, including ones funded by NIH. Yet approval of therapeutic mushrooms by America's FDA is slow. Vetting is rigorous, drug research is lengthy and costly, plus pharmaceutical companies develop only those that would be profitable. Medicinal mushrooms are mainly available in the United States as dietary supplements that claim to maintain optimal health and ward off infections.

Table 5. Summary of Fungi with Therapeutic Benefits.

Fungus	Boosts Imune System	Anti-cancer	Anti-biotics	Brain Support	Anti-inflammatory	Reduces Cholesterol	Anti-diabetic
Maitake	+	+	+	+		+	+
Turkey tail	+	+					+
Reishi *Ganoderma lucidum*	+	+	+	+	+	+	+
Lion's mane *Hericium erinaceus*	+	+	+	+			+
Chaga	+	+	+		+		+
Birch polypore		+	+		+		
Tinder conk		+	+		+		
Artist's conk	+	+	+		+	+	+
Oyster mushroom *Pleurotus ostreatus*	+	+	+		+	+	
Chicken-of-the-woods		+	+		+		+
Red-belted polypore		+	+		+		+
Shiitake	+	+	+			+	+
Agarikon	+		+		+		
Cordyceps	+	+	+	+	+	+	+
Enoki	+	+	+	+	+	+	
Agaricus brasiliensis	+	+	+			+	
Split-gill mushroom	+	+	+		+		

Chang et al. 2012.
Marley 2009.
Patel and Goyal 2012.
Rogers 2015.
Stamets 2005.
Tang et al. 2016.

Benefits of medicinal mushrooms have peppered newspaper and magazine articles over the last few years. Social media have also helped promote healing mushrooms. Manufacturers tout them as superfoods. Turkey tail, reishi, shiitake, chaga, lion's mane, maitake and cordyceps have grown in popularity. Many people believe that fungal bioactive compounds offer a better natural alternative to chemically synthesized drugs. Shiitake and maitake taste fine as powders, but turkey tail, reishi and cordyceps are bitter — they may be taken as capsules or tinctures. Extracts from several mushroom varieties combine to have a greater health-promoting effect than a single species. Blends are multifunctional. Mushrooms are an 'in' thing at cafés and bistros, where they are added to coffees, teas, cacaos, shakes and chocolate bars. Actress Gwyneth Paltrow adds a mushroom extract to her morning smoothie. In 2018, Whole Foods Market listed mushroom products as their third fastest growing food category in the United States with medicinal mushrooms as a top food trend. Technavio (a marketing research company) predicted that the medicinal mushrooms market will grow by 4.55 billion dollars from 2020 to 2025, at a compound annual rate of 9.15 percent.

Several mushroom compounds regulate our immune systems.

Elderly people succumb to more infections because body defense mechanisms become less resilient with age. The Covid-19 viral pandemic brought home the vulnerability of Maine's elderly — 21% of its citizens are over sixty-five. Requests for immune-boosting mushroom products were so high during the April 2020 peak of the pandemic that several websites stated, "Due to high demand we are experiencing delays that will affect delivery." I had tried to order some. A head cold walloped me in mid-March. I had no Covid symptoms but all of my granny's remedies—plenty of sleep, chicken soup and a chest lathered with Vicks VapoRub™—failed. I eventually found turkey tail mycelium powder at my local wellness pharmacy. My cold vanished in a week. Turkey tail may have helped strengthen my immune system, yet I might have recovered without this mushroom product or experienced a placebo effect. I shall never know, but I became a convert of medicinal fungal supplements after I researched articles for this book.

Some American scientists worry about a current market hype of mycomedicine, because most data were obtained from lab experiments rather than human clinical trials. They also warn that the public need to be more cautious. A daily mushroom supplement that modulates your immune system over a long period may tip it out of balance or produce side effects such as heart disease.

Customers need to be savvy of mushroom product claims about concentrations and sources of medicinal polysaccharides (mycelium or fruit body). An independent review of nineteen different reishi neutraceuticals found that only 25% contained sufficient quantities of bioactive components to be effective. America's FDA allows manufacturers to state only that mushroom supplements have antioxidants that support immune systems. The American Herbal Products Association released label guidelines for fungal dietary ingredients, though product tags may disguise or misdirect customers. Grain substrates raise total polysaccharide content of mycelium products. Milled powders may have fewer bioactive ingredients compared with tinctures, because some therapeutic components are extracted only by alcohol.

Nevertheless the American public seems to be convinced.

Mushroom Cosmetics

Mushrooms contain natural beauty boosters that heal and protect skin as well as hair and nails. Health-giving compounds from eighteen different mushrooms are incorporated into lotions, oils, creams, serums and shampoos.

Chitosan, extracted from fungal cell walls, is widely used in cosmetology as a gel-forming antibacterial agent with moisturizing properties. Mushroom antioxidants play an essential role in skin repair and maintenance. Birch polypore produces antibacterial plus anti-inflammatory agents that calm irritated skin and address uneven tones. Cordyceps contains a substance that improves circulation, an added bonus for skincare products. Snow mushrooms excel at holding water and plump up your skin to make it silky. Schizophyllan, a polysaccharide of split-gill mushrooms, regulates cell responses to environmental stressors that might influence skin-aging. The Japanese have incorporated reishi into rejuvenating skincare products since the 1980s, but they hit the American market only after the turn of the century. Mushrooms are a good source of selenium, zinc and kojic acid, three functional ingredients of toiletries. Selenium in hair conditioners treats dandruff, seborrheic dermatitis and psoriasis. Zinc has antibacterial and anti-inflammatory properties that control acne. Kojic acid lightens skin. A yellow carotenoid pigment of chanterelles is added to suntan lotions to protect skin from harmful UV rays. Mushrooms are a fad in hair products, because their vitamins and minerals stimulate scalp follicles plus their glucans protect hair fibers and smooth tangles.

An April 2020 MarketWatch report stated that ‘shroom’ cosmetics are a major driver in the mushroom product boom.

Table 6. American Cosmetics with Healing Mushroom Ingredients.

Product Name	Mushroom	Advertised Functions
Aveno Positively ageless defoliating cleanser	Shiitake	Removes dirt, oil and makeup. Fights signs of ageing.
Osmia Organics Brightening facial serum	Shiitake	Makes skin bright and luminous.
CV Skin Labs Body repair lotion	Reishi	Heals wounds and fights inflammation.
Origins Mega-mushroom skin relief face mask	Reishi	Helps soothe irritated, inflamed skin.
Moon Juice Spirit dust	Reishi	Supports immune system.
Moon Juice Beauty shroom plumping jelly serum	Snow mushrooms	Hydrates and enhances skin elasticity.
Volition Water serum	Snow mushrooms	Hydrates and minimizes facial pore size.
Root Science Organic face mask	Chaga	Helps soothe irritated inflamed skin.
Murad Invisiblur perfecting shield	Mushroom peptides	Diminishes fine lines and wrinkles by helping regulate collagen and elastin.
Mádara Cosmetics, Boost –Three-minute growth boost and hair serum	Chanterelles	Supports a healthy scalp, boosts hair growth and protects fibers.
Groh® shampoo	Reishi	Restores hair growth.
Florasis Cordyceps care make-up remover cream	Cordyceps	Nourishing skin.

Devash and Norris 2018.
Hartfield 2021.
Mádara Cosmetics 2020.
Wu et al. 2016.

Psychedelic Mushroom Therapy

The United States government froze research funds on therapeutic uses of mushroom hallucinogens in the 1960s, after transcendental drugs were adopted by a widespread youth counterculture.

Psilocybin, a mind-altering alkaloid, is produced by roughly 200 mushroom species from fourteen different genera. One hundred and sixteen are in the genus *Psilocybe*. Several species grow in New England with blue-staining on their stalks, though they are difficult to identify. Psilocin (the active product of psilocybin) acts on brain receptors used by serotonin, a neurotransmitter that regulates mood, social behavior, libido, appetite, sleep, temperature, heart rate and other body functions. Psilocybin and its derivative psilocin are listed as schedule 1 drugs in America, along with opium and heroin. Cultivation of mushrooms that contain psilocybin and psilocin are banned in the United States. Illegal possession in Maine may mean a year in jail or a $2,000 fine. You may also receive a five-year prison sentence or a $5,000 penalty for selling them in Maine.

America is currently in a renaissance — psilocybin therapy to treat mental health conditions and addiction is once more accepted and validated. This may be due, in part, to an opioid crisis that swept across the country as well as a rise in depression, suicide and veterans' post-traumatic stress disorder. In clinical psilocybin trials at low doses, positive effects (with minimal safety concerns) were observed for depression, anxiety, obsessive compulsive disorder plus schizophrenia.

From 2004 to 2008, UCLA Medical Center performed double-blind tests to determine whether psilocybin reduced anxiety in terminal cancer patients. Those given the drug showed a significant decline in distress compared with those who received a placebo. An added bonus was that psilocybin acted within hours with benefits that lasted months. Traditional antidepressants take weeks to kick in and have to be taken each day. The FDA granted psilocybin a breakthrough therapy designation in 2019 to accelerate trials of its effectiveness as an antidepressant. Other studies demonstrated that psilocybin reduced end-of-life fear in terminal patients, induced a sense of release, retrieved memories and promoted peaceful introspection.

Research groups at several American universities have investigated psilocybin's ability to beat alcohol, nicotine, cocaine and opiate dependence. Some success has been reported with relatively small data sets (hundreds vs. thousands of participants), though programs are controversial.

Anecdotal accounts suggest that 'shroom' experiences may change a person and have long-term benefits. People have reported that psilocybin allowed them to blend physical, mental and spiritual worlds to attain peace. Debates about recreational use of psilocybin continue in America, though non-addictive some people do have adverse reactions such as anxiety and panic attacks or disturbing hallucinations.

In 2000, Johns Hopkins was granted permission to conduct a small trial (thirty-six people) on the effects of psilocybin on healthy volunteers, versus those given a placebo. Two or three doses were administered at two month intervals. Experiments were carefully monitored, because certain individuals are more susceptible to psilocybin than others. Professionals were assigned to each participant to prepare and guide them through each session as well as follow-up consultations. Sixty percent of volunteers who received psilocybin reported they had a mystical encounter with an increased sense of well-being that lasted up to fourteen months. A few psilocybin recipients announced their experiences were the most significant of their lives with positive results in mood, behavior and social interactions. They also became more aware and appreciative of nature.

An article in *Nature* magazine (November, 2021) reported that adults who microdosed on mushroom psychedelics had lower levels of anxiety and depression, as well as increased motivation.

Oregon legalized psilocybin mushrooms for medicinal purposes in 2020 and decriminalized possession of small quantities of all drugs. A group, Decriminalize Maine, seeks to follow the Oregon model and promote the healing properties of psychedelics such as psilocybin mushrooms. In April 2021, the Maine Psilocybin Services Act (LD 1582) was introduced to the state legislature. Subsequently a bill was passed in the House of Representatives that would reduce possession of scheduled drugs to a fine rather than incarceration, but the bill was shot down in the Maine Senate. Dirigo Psychedelic Society, based in Portland Maine, holds monthly meetings. Their mission is to create a safe space to discuss how psychedelics can benefit people both spiritually and therapeutically.

WHO'S GROWING MUSHROOMS

Global Production

Commercial mushroom cultivation is booming because people are eating more of them. From 1978 to 2012 global mushroom consumption increased twenty-seven fold. Most of this increased production was from Europe and Asia-Pacific. China was a major player, with three quarters of global output (forty million tons). The worldwide mushroom market is predicted to expand to $86 billion by 2025.

North American Production

Over 97% of mushroom sales in the United States are of *Agaricus bisporus*, white buttons and brown variants — baby bellas (crimini) and full-grown portabellas that have the strongest taste. Domestic production steadily increased from 2010 to 2017 by seven fold (USDA data). Retail sales of *Agaricus* grew by 5.5% in 2018, which outpaced total produce (at 3%). The Mushroom Council (a branch of the USDA) reported that sales maintained an upward trajectory between 2019 and 2020 in all fifty regions.

Pennsylvania and California are our two largest mushroom producers. Sixty percent of all white buttons cultivated in the United States come from Pennsylvania. Since 1937, they have sprouted in trays filled with dank composted manure in tunnels of a former limestone mine in Worthington, Armstrong County. They are also propagated in mushroom houses at sixty-one farms in Chester County. Some Italian, Quaker and Mexican families are fourth generation mushroom farmers.

A specialty mushroom market has also soared in America — sales between 2003 and 2015 more than doubled (USDA data). In 2016, production was valued at $95 million, a 30% jump from the previous year. This surge continued. From 2019 to 2020, specialty mushrooms increased in dollar and volume sales by 31%.

Commercial Cultivation in Maine

A commercial movement is underway in Maine to meet an increased demand for local mushrooms. Farm-to-table restaurants are popular in our state and mushrooms are a fast-growing crop that may be cultivated indoors year-round. Maine farmers have focused on specialty mushrooms and left *Agaricus* cultivation to large out-of-state producers.

Some of Maine's mushroom farmers use indoor growth systems along with log cultivation or outdoor beds. They practice sustainable techniques. Organic waste (sawdust, woodchips, grain hulls, composted animal manure, straw or corn cobs) go in, edible mushrooms come out. Spent growth substrate is sold to farmers for crop fertilization because it is loaded with nitrogen. Reported USDA sales for Maine mushrooms were negligible from 2002 to 2015, less than $8,000 per year, but rose sharply in 2016 and reached $1.2 million the following year. Most of this increase appeared to be due to a ramp up of farm output, since numbers of producers barely doubled and price per pound rose only slightly over this period. Mousam Valley Mushrooms in York County shipped 5,000 pounds of fresh mushrooms per week to retail outlets at the start of 2018 and doubled that by the end of the year. Sales continued to rise in 2019 and 2020. Erik Lomen, of Maine Cap N' Stem, argued that Maine's mushroom production is underestimated because most were cultivated on small holdings — the Mushroom Council report only on producers who supply over half a million pounds per annum. Hannaford and Shaw's supermarkets primarily stock *Agaricus* produced out of state, but carry a selection of Maine-grown varieties. Specialty stores and neighborhood organic markets across Maine offer a much larger selection of local fresh mushrooms. Whole Foods' display in Portland makes fungi fanatics drool.

Oyster Creek Mushroom Company in Damariscotta has been in business since 1989. I took my students on a field trip there in 2009, when I taught eleventh and twelfth grade science at the Deck House School in Edgecomb. At that time, the Damariscotta farm grew mushrooms indoors in trays and bag cultures or outdoors on tree stumps and stacked logs.

Packets of a dried wild mix lay on a counter and we learned that ten pounds of fresh mushrooms were required to make one pound of dried product. Owner, Dan Holden, took us on a tour of his property. The kids gawked at shiitake poking out of oak logs and begged to bring back a bag of mycelium to flush (grow a crop of) fresh mushrooms at school.

Mousam Valley Mushrooms is Maine's largest mushroom supplier. The Sharood family renovated a dairy barn in 2012 at Springvale, York County, to run their operation. Back then, Oyster Creek Mushroom Company in Damariscotta, Shiitake Farm in Rumford and a dozen wild foragers were their only competition. John Sharood's goal was to nourish New England with fresh, organic, culinary varieties year-round. Son Robert maintained pure cultures of fungi to inoculate bags of growth substrate. They subsequently switched to buy ready-made mycelium blocks or inoculated logs to save labor and time. A Maine Institute of Technology grant funded

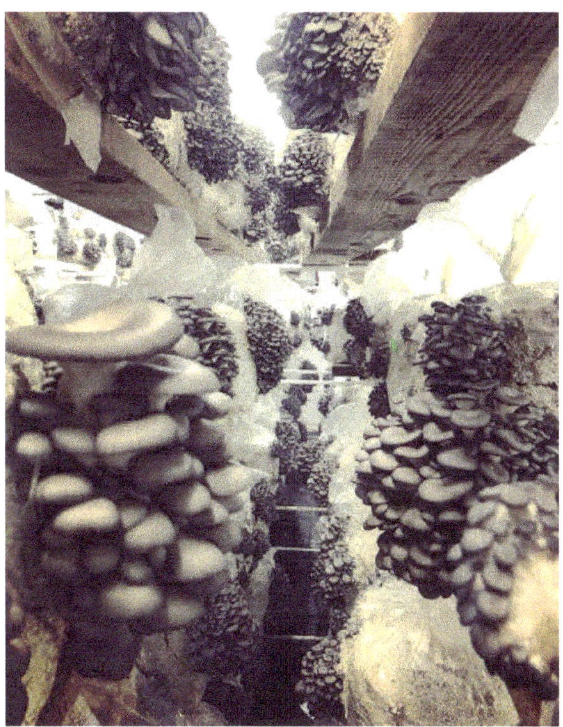

Italian oysters for Hannaford and Whole Foods supermarkets. (Courtesy of Mousam Valley Mushrooms.)

them to develop computer software that controlled temperature, humidity, light and airflow in special growth rooms. Oyster mushrooms develop in twenty-one days, shiitake take only seven to ten. Fresh mushrooms are harvested, packed and delivered within forty-eight to seventy-two hours in order to prolong shelf life. Mousam Valley Mushrooms' current facility (of two converted barns) has a capacity to produce 30,000 pounds. They cultivate a dozen varieties. Shiitake are the most popular. Italian oysters, lion's mane plus a forest medley are also good sellers. Spent growth substrate is sent to Maine farms to use as a compost/soil topper. A fleet of vans delivers Mousam Valley's produce to supermarkets and organic neighborhood stores from Delaware to Canada's Maritime Provinces. John Sharood's initial target group was millennials, because they tend to pay more for local, organic, high-quality products. The Springvale Company offered educational mushroom programs to Maine high schools, colleges, plus the University of New England at Biddeford. "Our goal is to reach $5 to $8 million in sales in five to ten years," John Sharood told *Mainebiz* in 2017. Leftover mushroom stems and pieces are made into a bisque (his mother's recipe) or bulk packed. John hopes to work with more institutions to use broken mushroom bits. A representative of University of Maine Dining said, "We're proud to feature Springvale, Maine's own Mousam Valley Mushrooms. They're beautiful and delicious."

North Spore cultivates spawn (mycelium growing on a food substrate) as well as mushrooms in southern Maine. This urban agriculture business was founded in 2014 by Jon Carver, Matt McInnis and Eliah Thanhauser, buddies from their student days at College of the Atlantic. All were interested in botany, mycology and agriculture. They converted a 500-foot Westbrook garage to grow edible mushrooms plus a range of medicinal polypores. Jon, a mycology graduate, maintained a spore bank of different strains to inoculate a variety of growth substrates. The company's initial goal was to provide fresh high-quality mushrooms to restaurants, food stores and cooperatives within a twenty mile radius. In 2016, North Spore moved their operation into Dana Warp Mill in Westbrook to accommodate their growing business. They supplied over seventy-five restaurants with fresh mushrooms before the Covid-19 pandemic hit — mostly in Portland, though they had customers from Mount Desert Island to Boston. North Spore was also a regular vendor at farmers markets in Brunswick, Portland, Kennebunk, Saco and York. This Maine mushroom business won a Gorham Savings Bank business competition in 2018 as well as a Greenlight Maine entrepreneurial pitch contest. North Spore convinced judges that increasing consumer interest and their new e-commerce platform would help increase sales. Prize money bought two labor-saving devices, a large autoclave to replace small pressure cookers that sterilized growth substrate and an automated packing machine to keep up with demand. Winnings also enabled North Spore to explore educational avenues to bring mushrooms to the public. Their mission: "To make the world of mushrooms more accessible to all, fostering innovation and collaboration to improve tomorrow." They offer classes, instructive videos, books and mushroom walks. North Spore still grows fresh mushrooms on site, but these are primarily for research and development. Most of their current business is to provide pure cultures, spawn and cultivation supplies to home-growers, gardeners and small farms. Sales boomed during the coronavirus pandemic of 2020. Matt McInnis told the *New York Times* that supplies to first-time growers were up 400% from the previous spring.

Three types of spawn are available for large commercial cultivators and home-growers. Plug spawn (mycelium growing on wooden dowels) to inoculate hardwood logs incubated outdoors, sawdust-spawn (an alternative log inoculum) and grain-spawn. Shiitake, lion's mane, oyster mushrooms and wine caps are popular varieties for outdoor beds. Simple spray-and-grow kits for kitchen counters are hot items on North Spore's website. They also supply them to Maine nurseries such as Skillins and Broadway Gardens. Lion's mane is a top seller. Their white pom-poms bust out of a box in just a few weeks. North Spore also takes online orders for dried mushrooms, tins of chaga tea, plus a range of health-promoting fungal powders and bottled tinctures.

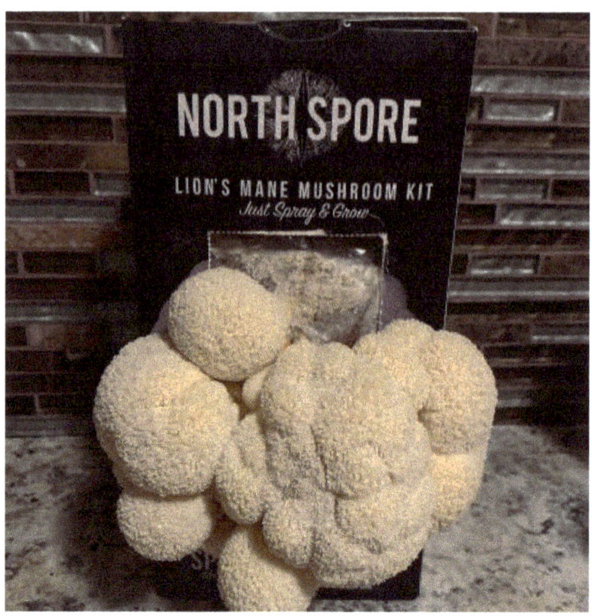

Lion's mane growth kit. (Courtesy of Northspore)

Maine Cap N' Stem Mushroom Company produce dense mycelium blocks of special varieties at a former wool mill in Gardiner — a vast industrial space shared with a whoopie pie bakery. Christopher Campbell and Erik Lomen started Cap N' Stem in 2014. They switched a few years ago from flushing mushrooms to selling growth kits of mycelium to farmers. Erik gave me a tour. I grinned as a young guy whizzed by on a skateboard to get to another part of the building. We approached a set of pallets piled high with ginormous sacks of wood pellets. Eric informed me that they had conducted numerous trials over the years to develop a specific blend of substrate additives to grow each mushroom species. They switched from a regular high tannic sawdust that had to be composted outdoors, to red oakwood pellets. These are conditioned with nitrogen-rich, non-genetically modified soybean or cotton seed hulls, or wheat middlings. The resultant carbon to nitrogen ratio depends on which mushroom variety they want to grow. A thrum of machinery grew louder as we strolled toward another part of the factory. We walked up a narrow metal staircase to view growth substrate churning in a rotating ribbon mixer. Down below an automated system weighed out portions, added water and dispensed the mix with a sudden whoosh into clear, high-strength, plastic bags. Batches were steam-sterilized in a mammoth stainless-steel autoclave, then cooled and inoculated with mushroom spawn in a super-sterile restricted lab. Cap N' Stem have maintained their own spore bank since 2019. Their in-house breeding program scales up production from lab cultures to bags of grain spawn to six-pound master bags to ten-pound blocks.

I then followed Erik into a climate-controlled incubation room where towering floor to ceiling shelves held closely spaced blocks of actively growing mycelium. Filter patches allow a fungus to breathe (oxygen goes in, car-

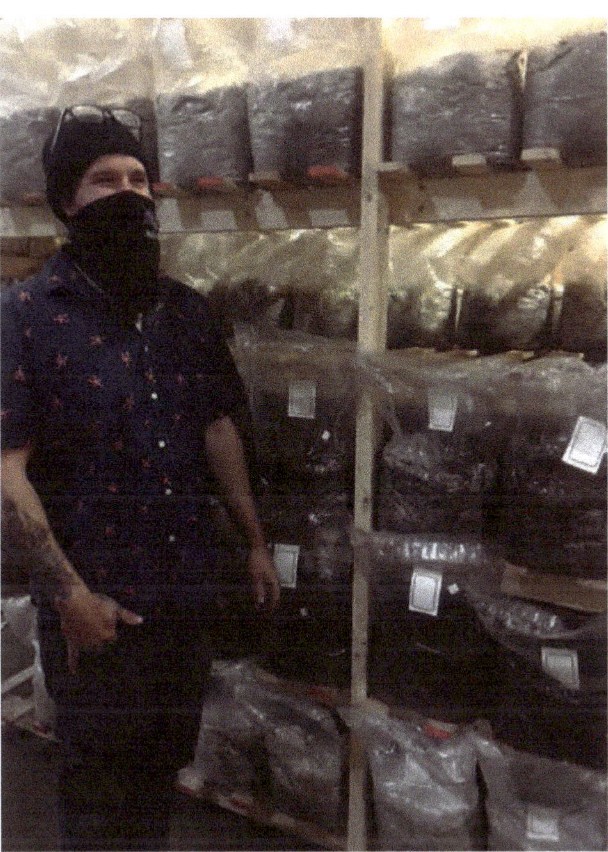

Erik Lomen by shelves of incubating mycelium blocks at Maine Cap N' Stem. Hilary Bartlett.

bon dioxide comes out). Immense fans whirled to maintain an even temperature of 66°F. "These blocks are really high in moisture content and nitrogen," Erik said. "So the organism that's running through it is just vigorous as all hell and heats up. If you're not careful they'll overheat." Incubation times varied from one to three weeks depending on species. Fully-aged blocks were firm and full of condensation. Growth was halted by transferring them to a chilled storage room (34°F). Dormant blocks of mycelium are shipped out in refrigerated vans to customers from Portland, Maine, to Portland, Oregon, as well as Canada. "Most of the farms we work with know how to flush them," Erik said. "They have a protocol for every one of them." Home-growers may order a single mycelium block (with instructions) from Cap N' Stem's website. Shiitake and oysters are the most popular. They are also their fastest growers. Maitake and reishi take a long time to colonize a ten-pound block of substrate. The Gardiner nursery also cultivates mycelium for lion's mane, namekos, pioppinos, chestnuts, and beech mushrooms. A pallet of 160 blocks produces on average 300 to 400 pounds of mushrooms, but yields may be much higher. Maximum capacity per incubation room is 8,000 blocks. Cap N' Stem have doubled their production each year since 2014.

Bountiful Mushroom Farm cultivates gourmet varieties in a warehouse wedged between a pool hall and railway tracks on the outskirts of Portland. They are part of Maine's effort to supply produce from farm-to-table year-round. The three farmers experimented for two years until they worked out how to efficiently flush different varieties from bags of sterile sawdust mixed with wheat straw in climate-controlled grow tents. By 2014, they harvested 150 pounds of mushrooms a week. They supplied lion's mane, shiitake, plus blue and golden oyster mushrooms to twenty-five of Portland's upmarket restaurants before the Covid-19 pandemic struck. Bountiful Mushrooms also sells their produce to the public through Alewive's Brook Farm.

Maine Mushroom Company is a small family-owned business based in Augusta. They grow organic gourmet mushrooms for high-end local restaurants and grocery stores, as well as farmers markets in Augusta, Hallowell and Lewiston. Maine Mushroom Company worked with Lost Kitchen's roadside-stand, launched in late March of 2020, to provide neighbors with fresh produce during the pandemic. The outdoor market in Freedom offered curbside Saturday morning pickup for people who ordered ahead. They often had 350 customers.

Andrew Dostie became hooked on videos about mushroom cultivation after he was laid off from a bakery during the Covid-19 contagion. He pitched the idea of a mushroom business to his uncle, Pat Bolduc, and B & D Family Mushroom Farm opened a retail store in January 2022 in Auburn, Maine. They have four growth rooms out back, where they currently propagate two varieties of oyster mushrooms and lion's mane. Andrew also bakes and their roasted mushroom/cream cheese spread tastes scrumptious on his freshly made bagels. Customers may also buy mushrooms in bulk or packets of dried ones, as well as cartons of mushroom soup or stew.

Lisa Jonassen and Lou DiSalvo run Island Mushroom Company from their property on Westport Island in Midcoast Maine. They cultivate mushrooms indoors on supplemented hardwood sawdust for customers within a sixty-mile radius. Lisa and Lou also sell their products at farmers markets in Brunswick, Falmouth, Greater Gorham and Wiscasset. Their booth displays quarts of fresh mushrooms, packets of dried shiitake nibbles plus a wild mix. Reishi tea bags blended with rooibos and orange peel are on offer as well as medicinal mushroom tinctures and powders (pre-seasoned or plain). The couple also have a line of Vegan Memorable Mushroom Burgers made with either shiitake or lion's mane.

Toshio Hashimoto, a first-generation Japanese immigrant, has operated a successful shiitake business out of Rumford for decades. He and his wife cultivate shiitake on oak logs, a traditional method in Japan. They run workshops out of their greenhouse for enthusiasts who want to learn how to grow them. Toshio's log-grown shiitake won a judge's award at the 2019 Common Ground Country Fair. People flocked to his booth to wolf down his famous deep-fried shiitake.

Sweet Relief Farm grow shiitake on red oak logs at their 400-acre homestead in Steep Falls, Standish. They sell them to local restaurants and have a booth at a local Farmers Market. Winslow Farm in Falmouth and Riverside Farm in North Yarmouth also offer log-cultivated shiitake.

Candice Hoydon of Oyster Creek Mushroom Company in Damariscotta reminisced about their shiitake operation when her husband, Dan, was alive. Their laying yard was in a shady spot near a water source on their property. They forced logs to fruit more often by drenching them in cold water overnight. "We were soaking a hundred logs a week to get to market," Candice said. Their logs produced four to five flushes before weather turned too cold, with a rest period of six to eight weeks between each soak.

In 2010, SARE (Sustainable Agriculture Research and Education) sponsored a five year project to cultivate shiitake on logs in New England. Participants included growers from Maine. Each learned basics of cultivation as well as forest management. A bulk of their work was carried out in winter when farm activities were minimal. Red oak gave better shiitake production compared with other hardwoods. Winter and spring yields beat those of spring and summer. A prolific log fruited for four or more seasons. Most labor (53%) was felling trees and cutting logs, with 32% for maintenance plus 15% for marketing and distribution. Greater efficiency was achieved by cultivators who had a well-designed growth yard. Forty-six percent of shiitake production was sold to restaurants with smaller amounts to farmers markets and grocery stores. Chefs paid ten to sixteen dollars per pound for log-grown shiitake, twice that of indoor flushes. Demands at local markets far exceeded an individual grower's supply. Net profits were obtained for two thirds of those who completed the project, with an estimated $9,000 return over five years. An indirect bonus was that thinning a tree stand for mushroom cultivation improved forest health.

Middle Earth Mushrooms produce log-grown shiitake, golden oysters and lion's mane at Seal Cove Farm on Mount Desert Island. Dominika and John Delmastro experimented for two years before they jumped into serious production. Customers order online for pick up at the farm or home delivery. Inoculated logs are soaked in an ice bath each night and left outside each day, which fools a fungus into thinking spring arrived and they fruit. Dominica and John built a greenhouse to extend their season but noted that mushrooms grown outdoors tasted better plus they have more vitamin D. The couple participated in a farm-drop program to help farmers from Washington and Hancock counties sell their produce during the Covid-19 crisis. Customers ordered online for a Thursday afternoon pickup at an outdoor stand in Floret, Somesville.

Lindsey and Teo Canino grow shiitake, oysters and wine caps on logs. They sell fresh mushrooms from their Milkweed Gardens farmstand in Sedgewick, Hancock County. You may also sample them at restaurants in Stonington and Blue Hill.

Bramble Hill Farm in Unity cultivates shiitake on logs. Plans are in the works to increase the size of this operation. They also grow oyster mushrooms indoors on certified organic straw from March through November. The farmers take advantage of ambient temperature to keep energy costs down and minimize their environmental footprint. "We are low tech," owner Suzanne Lametta said. "And depend a lot on seasonal temperature to determine which strains of mushrooms to grow." After her oysters flushed a few times indoors, Suzanne added that old growth substrate to her outdoor beds of woodchips used to grow wine cap *Stropharia* mushrooms. Bramble Hill Farm sells their fresh mushrooms at farmers markets in Belfast, Rockland and Deer Isle's night market. Suzanne told me that in 2020 they branched out to offer mushroom tinctures.

MannaFest Mushrooms sold oysters, shiitake, chestnuts and lion's mane from their Appleton farmstand and Guini Ridge Farmers Market in Rockport. The mushroom company set up a website in April 2020 to take orders for fresh ones. Home-growers may also order mycelium blocks and plug spawn from this online site.

The Mushroom Growers Newsletter (a monthly publication) listed only nine Maine cultivators in their 2020 spring issue, an underestimate, as they failed to include farmers who cultivate mushrooms along with other crops.

The Covid-19 pandemic directly affected Maine's commercial mushroom growers. Sales to restaurants went down. Sales at farmers markets and stores went up. Cultivators also shifted their focus to regularly update website information and fulfill increased numbers of orders made online.

Growing Mushrooms on Your Property

Mainers come from hardy stock and are proud of their self-reliance. As Maine humorist Tim Sample said, "We are independent as a hog on ice." Cultivating mushrooms on your property supports your family, sustains your local economy and reduces your carbon footprint. Northspore offers classes on growing mushrooms at Pineland Farms in Cumberland County. Online videos and blogs offer advice on how to grow them from spawn, or reach out to members of a local mushroom group and join Maine Mycological Association. Useful cultivation tips may also be found in books (Stamets and Chilton 1983, Stamets 1993, and Russell 2014).

In September, thousands congregate in Unity, Maine for the Common Ground Country Fair that celebrates organic agriculture and eco-friendly practices. A number of booths feature mushrooms. Maine Cap N' Stem and Maine Organic Farmers and Gardeners Association (MOFGA) held a mushroom cultivation workshop in 2017 at the fairgrounds, for farmers who wanted to diversify. Speakers provided information on how to grow different varieties on outdoor beds and indoor hoop houses.

Outdoor beds

You may choose to cultivate mushrooms outside on your property. North Spore has a helpful video. All you need is a sheltered place with dappled sunlight, waste resources, spawn and water. Perhaps you have a shady eastern or northern slope with minimal wind exposure? You may exploit a spot that is too wet and dark for most plants to grow or use natural topography, such as an indentation made by large roots of trees, as long as your garden hose will reach. Mushroom beds need to be watered especially during a drought. Choose varieties that you love to eat and experiment with different growth materials. Oyster mushrooms, forest namekos and almond *Agaricus* flourish on all types of organic debris. *Agaricus* species and shaggy manes prefer manure and wood blewits do well if debris is a bit more composted. What mushroom substrates are on your property? You may want to clear out a thorny thistle patch, recycle a mass of tenacious bamboo or dispose of a heap of dead leaves, but avoid composted wood mulch as this always contains competing fungal species. Mixed particle beds produce better results because mycelium needs oxygen to grow. A substrate that is too uniform in size will compact and may become anaerobic. Rural municipal dumps are a good source of uncontaminated woodchips. A tree removal business or a local lumber yard might deliver a truckload of wood waste in exchange for fresh mushrooms, plus a little compensation for the gas and time.

Namekos have a long history of cultivation in Japan, and have recently become popular in Maine. You can make nameko beds with layers of mixed hardwood chips inoculated with grain or sawdust spawn watered with a fine sprinkler (woodchips – spawn – water . . . repeat). Continue to layer until your bed is four to eight inches deep. Namekos are cold-loving, most growth occurs in fall. Water regularly to optimize success. Namekos are a standard ingredient in miso soup. They have a strong nutty flavor when thoroughly cooked. Their glossy amber caps have a silky texture, plus cap gelatins thicken sauces that complement poultry and red meat.

Oyster mushrooms were first cultivated in Germany as subsistence food after the First World War. They grow well on layers of compacted wheat straw (straw – spawn – water . . . repeat). Beds may be covered by a shade cloth as long as you leave a top space for ventilation.

Wine cap *Stropharia* flourish on beds of wheat straw or woodchips inoculated with plug or sawdust spawn. Their common name is garden giant because their caps grow as large as dinner plates. Flushes often exceed one family's needs. Young wine caps have a fine nutty taste and are good when grilled, sautéed or braised, older open ones lose their flavor.

Almond *Agaricus* prefers composted animal manure. These mushrooms should be inoculated in summer, because they love heat.

Log cultivation of shiitake

Production is initially labor intensive because you have to fell oak trees, cut logs and inoculate them. Leaf photosynthesis during summer ensures trees are busting with complex sugars by fall — an ideal mushroom substrate. Inoculation is performed at low temperature in late winter or early spring to minimize growth of fungal competitors. A trunk of four to five inches diameter has optimum sapwood per volume for shiitake spawn. Three to four foot lengths have a high potential for large numbers of flushes plus longer logs are more cumbersome. One inch holes are drilled four to six inches apart with a twelve millimeter bit or modified grinder. Rows with three to four inches between are staggered around a circumference. A greenhouse with a power source is ideal. A hand drill may be used outdoors. Sawdust spawn is added to each hole with a special tool, or wooden dowels

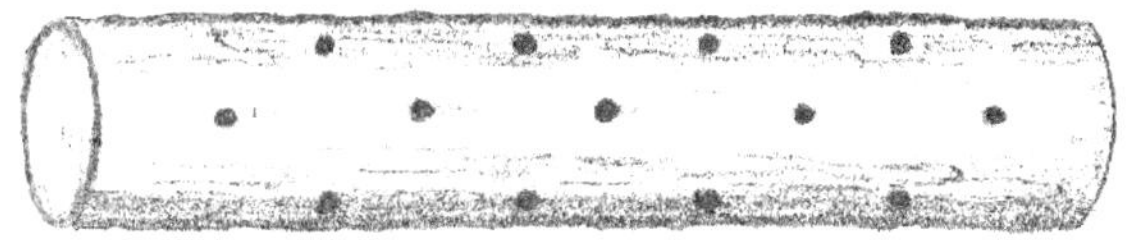

inoculated with mycelium (plug spawn) are tapped in place with a mallet. Three Maine companies sell shiitake spawn — North Spore, Oyster Creek Mushrooms and Mannafest Mushrooms. A dab of melted wax brushed on inoculated areas prevents bugs from crawling in to devour mycelium. Waxed log ends seal in moisture. A crockpot on low heat keeps wax molten if you have an electrical outlet, or melt the wax in a saucepan on a camp stove.

A tree canopy protects shiitake from direct sunlight. Logs stacked horizontally or laid in a zigzag pattern (of a split-rail fence) provide airflow and easy access to pick mushrooms. You may also lean logs at an angle against a shady barn wall. A laying yard near water is convenient. Chuck logs in a pond if they need to be hydrated during a dry spell or mist them overnight. Tarps should be replaced with a shade cloth after soaking. Logs need to be closely monitored in winter because they tend to dehydrate when air is dry.

Old blankets, draped over log stacks, shelter them during drying winter winds. Pallets allow logs to be close to a humid forest floor. Snow cover also provides great protection for inoculated logs.

Colonization takes five to twelve months in Maine. Performance depends on temperature and moisture. Shiitake fruit nine to fifteen months after inoculation, naturally occurring during spring and fall. One oak log produces a quarter to half a pound of mushrooms at each flush. They are harvested before they fully mature, when caps are still convex rather than flat. Shiitake should fill your basket to the brim by the second year. One log yields three to four pounds of fresh mushrooms over five years, about eight flushes. The first three are most prolific. My neighbors inoculated oak logs with shiitake plug spawn bought online. Fifteen months later they harvested their first flush.

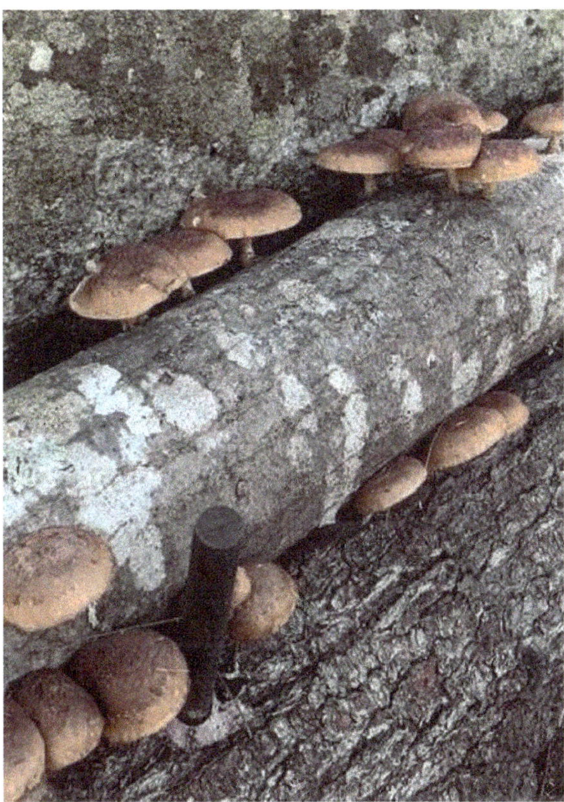

A shiitake flush on logs. Rita Arnold.

The Northeast Forest Mushrooms Growers Network is an online platform for shiitake cultivators, a site where like-minded mushroom enthusiasts share information and offer tips. Blind taste tests found that log-grown shiitake were superior to those cultivated on sawdust. Culinary professionals differentiated subtle differences in shiitake grown on various woods. Those on red oak had a meatier flavor, whereas those on sugar maple were milder and smoother. Lion's mane and oyster mushrooms also grow well on oak logs.

Mushroom cultivation on tree stumps

An advantage of growing mushrooms on stumps is that intact tree roots continue to suck up water. Recently cut stumps are preferable because older ones may already be colonized by fungi. Inoculation is ideally performed in early spring before air becomes saturated with spores. Oyster mushrooms, reishi, maitake and lion's mane thrive on stumps, but make sure you choose a variety that will grow on the type of wood you have chosen. Holes are drilled one inch inside peripheral sapwood on the sides of a stump. Wooden dowels coated with mycelium (plug spawn) are tapped in place then covered with wax. Or cut off a top section of wood, drill holes in the fresh surface, inoculate with plug spawn and replace the top (sandwich fashion). Another option is to cut a circular groove in bark with a chainsaw, then girdle the stump with rope soaked in a slurry of spores. Exposed rope is covered with wax. A combination of approaches maximizes your chance of success. Rain is sufficient to water inoculated stumps, though a good soak may coax a flush. Colonized wood will fruit for several years. Mushrooms may sprout continuously during a rainy fall.

Growing Mushrooms in Your Home

Maine has a brief outdoor growth season for vegetables. If you enjoy fresh produce from your garden, consider mushroom cultivation year-round in your home. North Spore offer simple spray-and-grow kits that fit on a kitchen counter. This is a great way for newbies, because these shoeboxes of mycelium are ready to be watered with results in just a few weeks.

Indoor tub cultivation

You may scale up to cultivate mushrooms in tubs. North Spore sells spawn and bags of growth substrate, plus their videos of tub cultivation have easy-to-follow instructions. First-time home growers often start with oyster mushrooms on pasteurized manure in a large (fifty to seventy quart), clear plastic, storage bin with a lid. Sterility is a key to success — invisible contaminants hang out everywhere, plus air conditioners and fans waft mold spores through your home. All materials including hands and forearms need to be sterilized with rubbing alcohol (seventy percent) to prevent contamination. Ventilation holes (two inches diameter) are cut into a tub because mycelium needs oxygen to grow. Holes plugged with Poly-fil™ provide sufficient gas exchange. Oyster mushrooms require low light levels to fruit. The bottom half of your tub must therefore be painted black to ensure that fruit bodies grow up towards light. The inside of a tub plus the lid must be thoroughly sprayed with alcohol and air-dried to remove contaminants before inoculation. A thin layer of grain spawn is sprinkled over the bottom of a tub. A bag of pasteurized growth substrate is squeezed to expel a few drops of liquid. This confirms a correct moisture content. The growth substrate is then scattered on top. Dry substrate may be sprayed with a mist of sterile (boiled) water after you spread it out. Spawn and substrate continue to be layered lasagna style. The lid must be resprayed with alcohol before your tub is sealed and incubated at room temperature.

Condensation on a cover is a good indicator of a healthy colony. Teensy, immature mushrooms (pins) form on top after two weeks. A one- to two-inch layer of coco coir (a hydroponic growth medium) is spread on top and saturated with sterile water. A spritz once or twice a day provides enough moisture for fruit bodies to form. Then voila! Your mushrooms have flushed. Secondary flushes take longer and produce fewer mushrooms. Leftover substrate may be added to your compost pile. *Agaricus* and shaggy manes also grow well in tubs.

MADE IN MAINE

Chaga Beer

Craft breweries have jumped onboard Maine's mushroom bandwagon to produce beers containing chaga, a woody polypore that boosts immune systems. Chaga rounds out flavor in ale to impart a slightly bitter tang similar to hops. I took a trip to Portland and stopped by Lone Pine Brewing Company to try their chaga stout. My seat at a picnic table overlooked a courtyard adjacent to a tasting room. A menu informed me that their dry chaga stout aged on vanilla beans was balanced to be dry, sweet and powerful. I popped open a chilled can and took a sip. "Most people don't know what chaga is," barmaid Erin said, "but they're willing to try it and like it when they taste it. And customers who love antioxidants are excited about it because chaga is packed with them." This brand was introduced in 2016 on draft and in cans. North Spore of Westbrook provides foraged chaga. Lone Pine Brewery supplies their chaga-infused beer to Maine taverns, restaurants and retail stores. The Portland brewery also services Boston.

Frosty Bottom Brewing of Belfast offers a porter brewed with chaga. What started out as a hobby among friends in 2014 turned into a community-supported business five years later (based on a farm shares model).

Ambition Brewing of Wilton makes a chaga English bitter in their 'Spottah T.E.A.' series of British ales. The business was founded in 2018 by two home-brewers who wanted to produce artisanal beers on a commercial scale.

Gruit Brewing Company at Urban Farm Fermentary in Portland offers an English-style mild beer with chaga as well as a dry chaga stout with dark chocolate notes. This brewery also adds medicinal reishi and lion's mane mushrooms to their beers.

Chaga Syrup and Teas

I spoke to Justin Wood when he came to grade my driveway. He taps maple trees in spring to make syrup at his Sweetwoods Farm in Newcastle. Justin reserves some batches to infuse with chaga in late fall to early winter. He sustainably harvests chaga from birch trees on his property when weather turns cold. Chunks are naturally dried and ground into smaller pieces. These are sealed in a porous bag that is steeped in five gallons of maple syrup for four or more hours at 190°F. The resultant dark syrup is then cooled and bottled. Justin's customers enjoy its woodsy flavor, plus chaga has healing powers.

White Cap Coffee out of Portland obtains chaga from North Spore to brew a health-promoting tea. Bar Harbor Tea Company also sells packets of sustainably harvested ground chaga.

Mushroom Dyes

Mushrooms are rich in tannins that make colorfast dyes for textiles and paper. Interest in natural eco-friendly stains has grown because industrial textile dyes account for 20% of global water pollution. Mushroom coloring agents were first developed in the 1970s in southern California. Protein fibers of wool accept mushroom dyes more readily than cellulose-based cotton or paper. Caps and stems are chopped up, mashed and simmered in spring water. Wool skeins are steeped in the mushroom teas. Inorganic substances, mordants, fix dyes to fibers to improve color fastness. An alkaline ammonium solution works well with most mushroom species. A mordant may change an original dye color. Cream of tartar may be used with a mordant fixative to help distribute a dye more evenly.

Ann Williams of Stonington, Maine, has displayed her colorful selection of mushroom-dyed wool skeins at presentations throughout the state. She steeps her yarn with mushroom teas in a three to one ratio (twelve ounces of foraged mushrooms to four ounces of wool). Decomposing specimens produce better results. A longer boil gives a more intense shade. Freezing mushrooms or chlorinated tap water also alter tints. Teas made from Dyer's polypore and lobster mushrooms require less fresh product.

Dyer's polypore produces a range of rich earth hues with different mordants.

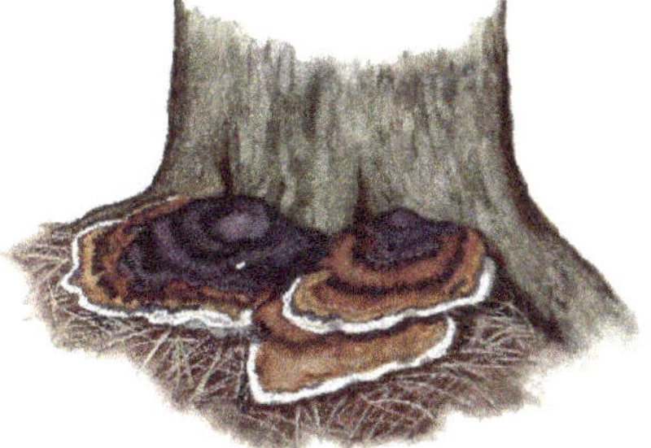

Dyer's polypore, *Phaeolus schweinitzii*.

Table 7. Coloring Yarn with Dyer's Polypore.

Mordant	Resultant Color
ammonia	orange
ammonia/copper pot	deep green
ammonia/iron pot	red rust
salt water	brilliant yellow

Spahr 2009.

Dezeen magazine's April 2020 issue reported on research of eco-friendly mushroom dyes carried out by Circular Union, a multi-skilled cross-industry collective. The company's founder, Mariah Wright, splits her time between her studios in Maine and Brooklyn, New York. Mariah's focus is on sustainable design elements. Her eyes sparkled when she spoke about her new range of mushroom dyes, Mush-Hues. In 2019, she worked with Maine foragers and mushroom farmers to develop a range of recipes for staining pine, a prolific resource in our state. Mariah's goal was to use renewable materials harvested only from Maine woodlands. Bags of mushrooms were steeped in vats of hot water to make rich teas. Various cooking and fermentation techniques were tested. Reclaimed pine boards were hand-colored, their soft porous fibers are well suited to absorb mushroom dyes. The final Mush-Hue collection has fifty colors for wood and textiles — from buttery yellows, grays and greens to pale pinks, plums and a soft shade of lilac.

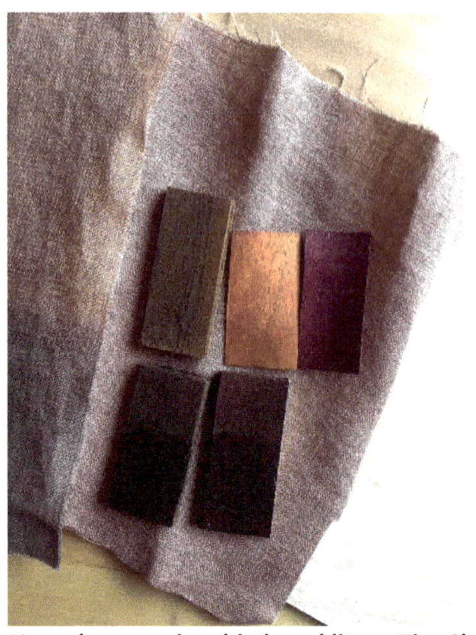

Mush Hues dyes on pine, birch and linen. Tim Clark. (Courtesy of Mariah Wright, Circular Union.)

MUSHROOM RECIPES FROM MAINE

Boothbay Crab-stuffed Mushrooms

(Chez Hilary, Boothbay Harbor)

Hors d'oeuvres

Ingredients

20 baby bellas (crimini)
4 oz. fresh Maine crabmeat
2 Tbsp. plain yoghurt (Swiss)
1 Tbsp. panko breadcrumbs
1 Tbsp. olive oil
1 tsp. Worcestershire sauce
¼ tsp. Old Bay Seasoning
1 Tbsp. lemon juice
Sea salt to taste
2 tsp. parsley, finely chopped
Parmesan cheese, grated for sprinkling
Paprika for sprinkling

Directions

1. Pop off stems. Brush caps with olive oil and place gill-side-down on a baking tray. Par-bake caps in a preheated 450° oven for about 5 to 7 mins until excess moisture has pooled onto the tray. Mop up expelled liquid with a paper towel and allow them to cool.
2. Reserve the crabmeat and mix the rest of the ingredients in a bowl. Gently fold in the crabmeat and mound the stuffing ½ inch over the top of each cap.
3. Sprinkle with cheese and paprika. Bake at 425° for 8 to 10 minutes.

Maine Wild Mushroom Dip

(Candice Hoydon of Oyster Creek Mushroom Company, Damariscotta)

Ingredients

¾ oz. Oyster Creek Maine Wild Mix (dried mushrooms)
1 Tbsp. olive oil
8 oz. cream cheese, softened
2 cloves roasted garlic, mashed
Fresh parsley or chives, chopped
Salt and pepper to taste

Directions

1. Reconstitute dried mushrooms in 2 cups of hot water for 30 minutes, drain and reserve liquid.
2. Rinse mushrooms with cold water. Press between paper towels to remove excess liquid and chop.
3. Sauté mushrooms in olive oil for a few minutes until soft.
4. Add soaking broth to the pan carefully avoiding any sediment at the bottom, and reduce until liquid is gone but mixture is still moist. Remove to a bowl and cool.
5. Add roasted garlic, cream cheese, herbs, plus salt and pepper.
6. Refrigerate before serving.

Hungarian Mushroom Soup

(A favorite at Bowdoin College)

Serves 8

Ingredients

6 oz. portabella mushrooms, sliced
12 oz. white button mushrooms, sliced
½ cup onion, diced
2 tsp. garlic, minced
4 Tbsp. butter or olive oil
4 tsp. sweet paprika
4 Tbsp. all-purpose flour
2¾ cups vegetable stock
1½ tsp. soy sauce
¾ cup milk
1 tsp. lemon juice
1 tsp. freshly ground black pepper
1 Tbsp. fresh dill, chopped
½ cup sour cream

Directions

1. Melt butter, add onions, mushrooms, paprika, garlic, half of pepper and half of dill. Cook on medium heat, stir often until onion and mushrooms are tender. Be careful not to burn. Do not break up mushrooms.
2. Add flour slowly and blend to make a roux. Cook 4 – 5 minutes.
3. Add stock, soy sauce and milk. Cook until thickened.
4. Add remainder of pepper and lemon juice and heat only to 160° or product will curdle.
5. Add sour cream before serving and adjust seasoning if required.
6. Use remainder of dill to garnish.

Portabella Mushroom Stuffed with Spinach and Gorgonzola

(Candice Hoydon of Oyster Creek Mushroom Company, Damariscotta)

Serves 4

Ingredients

4 medium sized portabella mushrooms
1 lb. fresh spinach, washed and chopped
1 medium onion, sliced
1 clove of garlic, finely chopped
2 tsp. olive oil
2 oz. Gorgonzola cheese
¼ cup water
1 salad bowl of mixed greens
Salad dressing, a balsamic vinegar and truffle oil mix.

Directions

1. Remove stems from mushrooms.
2. Heat 1 tsp. olive oil in a sauté pan and grill caps gill-side-down for 5 minutes. Turn caps over and cook with ¼ cup of water until liquid disappears.
3. In another pan, cook garlic and onions in 1 tsp. olive oil until onions are caramelized. Add spinach until wilted.
4. Stuff caps with onion and spinach mixture. Top with Gorgonzola cheese and cover. Heat a few minutes until cheese melts.
5. Serve stuffed mushrooms on a bed of greens tossed in truffle oil and balsamic vinegar.

Butternut, Sage and Oyster Mushroom Frittata

(Frank Giglio of Farm and Forage Kitchen)

Serves 4

Ingredients

2 generous portions of lard or ghee
1 large onion, diced
2 cups butternut squash, diced
1 heaped cup of oyster mushrooms torn into smaller pieces
5 – 6 kale leaves, stalk stripped away, greens chopped up
2 garlic cloves, minced
6 eggs
½ cup full fat milk
1 Tbsp. fresh sage, chopped
½ cup goat cheese cheddar, grated
Sea salt to taste.

Directions

1. Preheat oven to 350°.
2. Heat a #8 cast iron pan over medium heat. Melt the fat, add the onions and stir to combine. Heat for 2 minutes before adding squash. Cook for a few more minutes before adding mushrooms. Continue to cook, adding more fat if needed until the onions begin to caramelize and the squash browns up a bit too.
3. In the meantime, crack the eggs into a bowl along with the milk, salt, cheese and sage.
4. Once the squash are tender, turn off the heat and add the egg mixture, whisking gently before adding it.
5. Transfer the pan to the oven and bake for 15 min. or until center is firm to the touch.
6. Serve a wedge hot or cold with a side salad.

Baked Polenta with Shiitake

(Candice Hoydon of Oyster Creek Mushroom Company, Damariscotta)

Serves 4

Ingredients

1 lb. fresh shiitake
4 cups chicken stock
3 Tbsp. unsalted butter
1 cup yellow cornmeal
½ cup grated Parmesan cheese
4 oz. Fontina cheese
¼ cup olive oil
3 cloves garlic, minced

Directions

1. Bring chicken stock to boil in a heavy kettle. Add butter. Add cornmeal in a slow steady stream while whisking over low heat until very thick, about 15 minutes. Slowly whisk in Parmesan cheese.
2. Pour mixture into a buttered 8-inch pie dish and cool.
3. Preheat oven to 375°. Cover a baking sheet with parchment paper. Slice polenta into wedges, sprinkle with Parmesan and top with sliced Fontina. Place in oven for 20 minutes.
4. In a heavy skillet heat olive oil, add garlic and sauté for about 2 minutes. Add sliced shiitake and cook until mushrooms are lightly browned. Serve this mixture over baked polenta.

Twice Baked Potatoes with Maitake and Smoky Gouda

(Candice Hoydon of Oyster Creek Mushroom Company, Damariscotta)

Serves 4

Ingredients

4 large baking potatoes, baked until almost cooked through
2 oz. dried maitake mushrooms
6 oz. smoky Gouda cheese
2 oz. butter
3 – 4 slices of pancetta or bacon, diced

Directions

1. Bake potatoes in a 350° oven until almost cooked.
2. Cut potatoes lengthwise in half while still warm and scoop out flesh into a bowl without damaging their skins. Add half of Gouda cheese and all the butter to the warm potato filling and smash a little.
3. Reconstitute maitake mushrooms in hot water, just to cover, for 15 minutes. Drain, chop, put in a small skillet with pancetta or bacon. Sauté until bacon is crisp. Combine pan contents with potato mixture.
4. Scoop mixture back into potato skins. Top with remaining Gouda and bake again at 350° until hot, 12 to 15 minutes.

Mushroom Kale Bread Pudding

(Roberta Bailey, writer for Maine Organic Farmers and Gardeners Association)

Serves 10

Ingredients

1 lb. loaf of crusty coarse bread cut into 1 inch pieces (12 cups)
10 Tbsp. olive oil (divided)
1½ lb. of mixed store-bought mushrooms
1 medium onion, finely chopped
4 cloves minced garlic
1 cup dry white wine
2 cups kale, thinly sliced
2 cups of Gruyère or Swiss cheese cut in strips
10 large eggs
2 cups of vegetable or chicken broth
1 cup of milk (or nondairy substitute)
3 Tbsp. whole grain mustard
Salt and freshly ground pepper

Directions

1. Heat oven to 350° with rack in the middle.
2. In a large bowl, toss the bread with 3 Tbsp. of olive oil and 1 tsp. of salt. Spread the bread on a baking sheet and bake for 10 minutes. Turn the bread and bake for another 10 minutes until golden brown.
3. Heat 4 Tbsp. of olive oil in a large frying pan. Add mushrooms, onions, garlic and ground pepper. Stir and cook until the mushrooms release their water (about 3 minutes). Continue to cook until water evaporates (6 - 8 minutes).

4. Add wine, stir and scrape the bottom of the pan to release brown juices. Add kale and stir until wilted. Remove from heat.
5. Coat a 9 – 13-inch baking dish with the remaining 3 Tbsp. of oil. Mix the bread and mushrooms together and spread in the greased baking dish. Layer half the cheese on top.
6. Whisk the eggs in a bowl, add broth, cream, milk and mustard. Pour the egg mixture evenly over the bread combination. Cover and refrigerate for 1 hour.
7. Bake at 350° for 45 minutes. Add the remaining cheese to the top and bake for another 15 minutes.
8. Remove from oven and cool for 15 minutes before serving warm.

Porcini Pork Tenderloin

(Candice Hoydon of Oyster Creek Mushroom Company, Damariscotta)

Serves 4

Ingredients

1½ to 2lb. pork tenderloin (fat and silverskin removed)
¾ oz. Oyster Creek dried porcini
½ cup flour with salt and pepper to dredge pork
1 – 2 shallots, chopped
1 clove garlic, chopped
½ cup wine or chicken broth
1 cup water of soaking liquid from reconstituted porcini
1 to 2 Tbsp. olive oil

Directions

1. Soak porcini in 2 cups of warm water for 15 – 30 minutes. Strain mushrooms and save soaking liquid. Press porcini between paper towels to remove excess liquid then chop.
2. Slice pork into ¼ inch medallions, dredge in flour salt and pepper, sauté in 1 Tbsp. of oil until golden, remove and set aside.
3. Using the same pan add remaining oil to sauté garlic, shallots and chopped porcini for 10 minutes.
4. Deglaze the pan with wine or chicken broth. Return meat and soaking liquid to the pan. Cook over low heat until sauce thickens.

Chicken-of-the-Woods Stir-fry

(Jean Wood, my Tai chi buddy from Edgecomb)

Serves 1.

Ingredients

1 cup chicken-of-the-woods, cut into 1 inch pieces
1 sprinkling smoked applewood sea salt
½ cup broccoli, chopped into 1 inch pieces
1 cup snow peas
½ cup asparagus, cut into 1 inch lengths
2 shallots, chopped
1 to 2 Tbsp. peanut or grapeseed oil
3 oz. chicken, cut into cubes
1 Tbsp. rice vinegar
1 Tbsp. fish sauce or 1 Tbsp. Tamari soy sauce
¼ cup white wine

Directions

1. Parboil snow peas and broccoli for 30 seconds, rinse in cold water and reserve.
2. Heat 1 Tbsp. olive oil in a wok until hot, add mushrooms and stir for 4 minutes. Sprinkle with salt and stir. Reserve.
3. Cook shallots. Add more oil if necessary and stir over a high heat for 1 minute.
4. Add broccoli and asparagus plus rice vinegar, fish or soy sauce and wine. Cook and stir for 2 – 3 minutes.
5. Add snow peas and precooked mushrooms. Stir for 1 minute and serve.

Mushroom Clam Sauce on Pasta

(Roberta Bailey, writer for Maine Organic Farmers and Gardeners Association)

Serves 4

Ingredients

1 lb. fresh portabella, porcini, crimini and shiitake, cleaned and chopped
1 qt. raw shelled clams or canned clams
½ lb. pasta (spaghetti, linguini or fettuccini)
3 Tbsp. of olive oil
2 Tbsp. of butter or more oil
1 small onion, finely diced
3 cloves of garlic, minced
½ cup white wine
1 Tbsp. fresh parsley, finely chopped

Directions

1. In a deep sauté pan, heat the oil and melt the butter. Sauté the onion for 2 – 3 minutes.
2. Add mushrooms and sauté until soft.
3. Add garlic and sauté for 2 minutes.
4. Add clams and cook until liquid is reduced to less than half.
5. Add white wine and simmer for 3 – 5 minutes.
6. Meanwhile cook your favorite pasta. Drain and toss with the contents of your pan.
7. Serve and garnish with parsley.

Venison Stew with Wild Mushrooms

(Frank Giglio of Farm and Forage Kitchen)

Serves 4

Ingredients

2 Tbsp. rendered lard
1 large onion, cut into large chunks
3 carrots, cut into thick rounds
4 large garlic cloves, minced
2 Tbsp. tomato paste
1 lb. venison shoulder or hind leg, cut into large chunks
2 - 3 quarts stock or water
2 oz. dried wild mushrooms (or 2 cups of fresh)
2 bay leaves
1 cup acorn meal
Sea salt to taste
1 – 2 tsp. chopped sage, thyme or rosemary

Directions

1. Heat a 4 – 5-quart Dutch oven over medium-high heat. Add the onion and carrots, stir to combine, sauté for a few minutes.
2. Stir in the garlic, cook until fragrant.
3. Stir in the tomato paste and allow it to cook for 3 minutes or so, stirring as needed to prevent burning.
4. Add venison followed by the stock, mushrooms and herbs.
5. Bring the liquid to a boil, partially cover, reduce heat to medium and slowly simmer for an hour or so, until meat is tender.
6. Add the acorn meal and cook for another 10 mins.
7. Season and serve.

CONCLUSIONS

I jumped into this book project because it tapped into all of my passions — mushrooms, biology, art and cooking. Though daunting, this task was also an adventure, as I met some fascinating people along the way.

Mushrooms are fruit bodies of fungi that support plant, forest and human health as well as our economy. Climate change has affected wild mushrooms. A slight rise in temperature may increase mushroom yields and extend a fruiting season, but adaptations in fungal metabolism appear to be species dependent.

Mushrooms are touted as superfoods because they are low in calories, sodium and cholesterol, yet loaded with antioxidants, vitamins and minerals, plus numerous species have medicinal powers. Ancient civilizations used mushrooms for healing as well as food, yet modern America has only recently caught on. Eleven medicinal mushrooms are routinely foraged in Maine, though most are bought as powders, capsules or tinctures. Mycotherapy is used to strengthen immune systems, improve energy, support cognitive function and increase longevity. Health-giving compounds from eighteen different mushrooms are incorporated into cosmetics with the goal of healing and protecting skin, hair and nails.

Experiments on shroom-based psilocybin to treat mental health conditions had shown promise in the 1950s, but the United States government froze research funds on this hallucinogenic drug after magic mushrooms became part of the hippie scene. This federal policy has recently changed and clinical trials of psilocybin to treat depression are currently underway. Psilocybin therapy may also reduce end-of-life fear in terminal patients and help beat addiction. A group called Decriminalize Maine wants to make the possession of small quantities of psilocybin (a schedule 1 drug) subject to a fine rather than incarceration.

Maine's mushroom mania has spread as fast as mycelium. We forage, grow and eat more. Maine cultivators have ramped up production to meet increased demand at restaurants, farmers markets and grocery stores. For decades Maine supermarkets carried only cultivated white buttons, but now sell a wide variety of fresh, locally-grown, specialty mushrooms and packets of dried wild ones. Chefs add them to sauces and creamy risottos, toss them in pastas, sprinkle them on pizzas or float them in clear broths. Shipments of mushroom spawn to small-time growers and farmers also shot up. Maine vendors delivered to customers all over the country as well as Canada.

Sales of fresh mushrooms, cultivation gear and spray-and-grow kits continued to rise despite the Covid-19 pandemic, in part, because more families resorted to cooking at home. A call for fungal supplements that boost immune systems also spiked during the coronavirus crisis. Maine's expanding mushroom industry incorporates healing species into locally-crafted beers, teas and maple syrups, plus a colorful range of eco-friendly mushroom dyes for wood has been developed. An upswing in sales of Maine mushroom kits even made the *New York Times*.

GLOSSARY

alkaloid – a nitrogen-based organic chemical compound of mushrooms that produces a physiological reaction in humans.
amadou – interior, spongy, flammable flesh of a tinder conk shelf mushroom.
amino acid – a primary constituent of proteins.
anaerobic – without oxygen.
antibiotic – a chemical produced by a microorganism that inhibits growth or kills other microorganisms.
antibody – a blood protein produced in response to foreign cells or substances that binds to a foreign agent (antigen).
antidote – a medicine to counteract a poison.
antioxidant – a substance that removes damaging oxidizing agents produced by cell metabolism.
autoclave – a device that sterilizes materials by killing contaminants with steam under pressure.

bioactive – a substance that causes a biological effect.
biocontrol – use of an organism to control pests.
biofilter – a filter made of biological components.
biofuel – a renewable energy source derived from living material (biomass).
brown rot – fungal decomposition of cellulose in plants and trees.

cellulose – a structural polysaccharide polymer of plant cell walls.
chitin – a fibrous polysaccharide that gives strength to fungal cell walls.
compost – a mixture of microorganisms and decaying material.
compound – a substance made up of atoms from two or more chemical elements.

conifers – trees that produce cones and have needles instead of broad leaves.
conk – a tough shelf or hoof-shaped fruit body of a fungus that grows on trees.
cytokines – proteins important in cell signals that manage an immune response.

deciduous – of a tree that sheds leaves annually in fall.
degenerative disease – a progressive loss of function in organs and tissues.
DNA – deoxyribonucleic acid, a self-replicating molecule that carries genetic information.

ecosystem – an environment where populations of organisms live and interact.
effluent – liquid waste or sewage discharged into a natural body of water.
enzyme – a protein of an organism that speeds up a chemical reaction at ambient temperature.
ergosterol – a fungal precursor of vitamin D.
eukaryote – organisms with cells that contain a distinct nucleus and other membrane-bound structures.

filamentous – composed of long, thread-like, fungal filaments (hyphae).
flora – flowering plants.
flush – to grow a crop of mushrooms.
forage – to search for food from nature.
fraction – a quantity of chemicals collected from a mixture by a separation process.
fruit body – a spore-producing organ of a fungus, such as a mushroom.

fungi – a kingdom of non-photosynthetic, eukaryotic organisms that absorb nutrients from their environment — yeasts, molds and mushrooms, (fungus – sing.)
fungicide – a chemical that kills fungi.

gene – a hereditary unit (sequence of DNA) that determines a characteristic of an offspring.
genus – a principal taxonomic group of species, (genera – pl.).
germinate – begin to grow.
glucans – polysaccharide polymers of fungi.
glycoprotein – a class of proteins that consists of carbohydrates bound to a polypeptide chain.

habitat – an environment where organisms live.
hallucinogen – a substance that causes hallucinations.
humus – an organic component of soil formed by decomposition of plant material.
hyphae – hollow fungal tubes that transport chemicals.

immune-regulatory – regulation of an immune system.
immune system – a body's defense system that differentiates between host and foreign cells or substances and provides the host with immunity.
inflammation – white blood cells and chemicals act to defend a body against foreign substances or cell injury.
interferons – proteins released by host cells that inhibit virus replication.

laying yard – an outside area for storing logs used for mushroom cultivation.
lectins – a class of fungal proteins bound to sugars.
lignin – a complex polymer in cell walls of trees or shrubs that makes them rigid and woody.

magic mushrooms – an informal term for hallucinogenic varieties.
microbiome – a community of microorganisms that inhabit a specific ecosystem.
mildew – a visible coating of fungal hyphae on an object.
mold – a fungus with microscopic fruit bodies, visible as a soft fuzzy growth to a naked eye.
mordant – an inorganic chemical that fixes a dye to a material.
mushroom – a spore-bearing fruit body of a fungus that is visible to a naked eye.
mutagen – an agent that permanently alters an organism's DNA.
mycelium – a fungal network of hollow, branched tubes (hyphae) that invades food sources.
mycology – the study of fungi.
mycomediation – the use of fungi to degrade contaminants in an environment.
mycomedicine – application of mushroom-derived compounds with health benefits.
mycorrhiza – a nutritional association of fungal hyphae with plant roots that benefits both partners.
mycotherapy – use of fungal extracts and compounds to promote health.

neurotoxin – a poison that disrupts a nervous system.
neutraceutical – a dietary supplement that supports human health.
nucleus – a membrane-bound organelle within a cell that contains genetic material, (nuclei - pl.)

parasite – an organism that lives on and damages another organism, (parasitic – adj.).
partial veil – tissue that conceals developing gills in the earliest stage of mushroom development.
pathogen – a microorganism that causes disease.

peptide – a short chain of amino acids, the building blocks of protein.
perennial – persists for years.
peroxidase – an enzyme that catalyzes the oxidation of a compound by a peroxide.
petri dish – a shallow, circular, lidded vessel that holds gelled, nutrient-rich, growth medium for microorganisms.
phenol – a chemical with a hydroxyl group linked to a benzene ring.
pheromone – a chemical secretion that triggers a physiological response in members of the same species.
photosynthesis – a process by which plants convert light energy into chemical energy for growth.
placebo – a harmless pill with no therapeutic effect, used as a control in testing new drugs.
polymer – a large molecule made up of repeating subunits bonded together.
polypore – a mushroom that expels spores from tubes on the underside of a cap or conk.
polysaccharide – a long chain carbohydrate polymer made up of bonded sugars.
polysaccharopeptide – a long chain carbohydrate bound to a protein peptide.
psychedelic – a psychic effect of a drug such as a hallucination.

rust – a fungal plant disease that forms rust-colored spots on leaves, shoots, stems and fruit.

shroom – an informal name for a mushroom, especially for hallucinogenic varieties.
smut – a fungal disease characterized by soot-like masses that form on plants, especially grasses.
spawn – an aggregate of mycelium on a carrier that is used to culture mushrooms on a new substrate.

species – a biologically discrete group that interbreeds and produces fertile offspring.
spore – a reproductive fungal cell that produces a new individual of the species.
statins – a group of drugs that reduce blood levels of fats, triglycerides and cholesterol.
sterilization – to kill off life-forms.
sterol – naturally occurring lipids (unsaturated steroid alcohols - waxy solids)
strain – a race of individuals within a species that share common genetic traits.
substrate – a food source for fungal growth.

terpene – a diverse class of unsaturated hydrocarbons in oils of fungi.
tincture – an alcohol/water extract of fungi.
triglyceride – a primary constituent of fats and oils.
tuber – a thick, tough, underground food reserve that produces a new organism.
tundra – a vast, flat, treeless, Arctic region where subsoil is frozen.

universal veil – tissue that envelopes and conceals an entire button mushroom in early stage of development.

vegan – a person who does not eat or use animal products.

white rot – a fungal disease that degrades lignin of trees and woody shrubs.
wilt – a disease that affects vascular systems of plants.

yeast – a single-celled fungus that ferments sugars.

MUSHROOM NAMES (common and Latin)

agarikon – *Laricifomes officinalis* (*Fomitopsis officinalis*)
almond agaricus – *Agaricus subrufescens*
angel wings – *Pleurocybella porrigens*
artist's conk – *Ganoderma applanatum*

baby bella – *Agaricus bisporus*
bear's head tooth – *Hericium americanum*
beech mushroom – *Hypsizygus tessellatus*
birch bolete – *Leccinum scabrum*
birch clinker – *Inonotus obliquus*
birch polypore – *Fomitopsis betulina* (*Piptoporus betulinus*)
black trumpet – *Craterellus cornucopioides*
blewit (wood blewit) – *Clitocybe nuda*

cèpe – *Boletus edulis*
chaga – *Inonotus obliquus*
chanterelle – *Cantharellus* spp. (Formal names for N. American sp. are under revision.)
chestnut mushroom – *Pholiota adiposa*
chicken-of-the-woods – *Laetiporus sulphureus*
comb tooth – *Hericium coralloides*
common ink(y) cap – *Coprinopsis atramentaria* (*atramentarius*)
cordyceps – *Ophiocordyceps* (*Cordyceps*) *sinensis*
crimini – *Agaricus bisporus*

death cap – *Amanita phalloides*
destroying angel – *Amanita bisporigera* (most common species in Maine)

Dryad's saddle – *Cerioporus* (*Polyporus*) *squamosus*
dyer's polypore – *Phaeolus schweinitzii*

enoki (golden needle) – *Flammulina velutipes*

false morel – *Gyromitra esculenta*
false tinder conk – *Phellinus tremulae*
fly agaric – *Amanita muscaria*
forest nameko – *Pholiota microspora* (*nameko*)

garden giant – *Stropharia rugosoannulata*
giant puffball – *Calvatia gigantea*
golden chanterelle – *Cantharellus* spp. (Formal names for N. American sp. are under revision.)
golden needle – *Flammulina velutipes*
golden oyster mushroom – *Pleurotus citrinopileatus*

hedgehog mushroom – *Hydnum repandum*
hen-of-the-woods – *Grifola frondosa*
honey mushroom (honey fungus) – *Armillaria mellea*
hoof fungus – *Fomes fomentarius*
horse mushroom – *Agaricus arvensis*

Italian (phoenix) oyster mushroom – *Pleurotus pulmonarius*

jack-o'-lantern – *Omphalotus illudens* (*olearius*)

king bolete – *Boletus edulis*

lilac-brown bolete – *Sutorius* (*Tylopilus*) *eximius*
lingzhi – (Chinese term for reishi) *Ganoderma lucidum* grows in Asia
lion's mane – *Hericium* species
lobster mushroom – *Hypomyces lactifluorum*

maitake – *Grifola frondosa*
matsutake – *Tricholoma magnivelare*
meadow mushroom – *Agaricus campestris*
milk(y) cap – *Lactarius* species
morel – *Morchella esculenta*

nameko – *Pholiota microspora*

oyster mushroom – *Pleurotus* species

parasol mushroom – *Macrolepiota procera*
pheasant's back – *Cerioporus* (*Polyporus*) *squamosus*
pigskin puffball – *Scleroderma citrinum*
porcini – *Boletus edulis*
portabella – *Agaricus bisporus*
puffball – of *Calvatia* and *Lycoperdon* genera

Ravenel's stinkhorn – *Phallus ravenelii*
red-belted polypore – *Fomitopsis pinicola*
reishi – *Ganoderma tsugae* grows primarily on hemlock in Maine, and related species are occasionally found on maple or oak.
Ganoderma lucidum is native to Asia and Europe.

saffron milk cap – *Lactarius deliciosus*
scaber stalks – *Leccinum* species
scotch bonnet – *Marasmius oreades*
shaggy ink cap – *Coprinus comatus*
shaggy mane – *Coprinus comatus*
sheep's head – *Grifola frondosa*
shiitake – *Lentinula edodes*
sickener – *Russula emetica*
snow mushroom – *Tremella fuciformis*

split-gill mushroom – *Schizophyllum commune*
stinkhorns – *Phallus* species
sulphur-shelf – *Laetiporus sulphureus*
sweet tooth – *Hydnum repandum*

tinder conk – *Fomes fomentarius*
tippler's bane – *Coprinopsis atramentaria*
truffles – *Tuber* species
turkey tail – *Trametes versicolor*

white button mushroom – *Agaricus bisporus*
wine cap Stropharia – *Stropharia rugosoannulata*
wood blewit – *Clitocybe nuda*

zombie fungus – *Ophiocordyceps unilateralis*

BIBLIOGRAPHY

Adimando, Stacey. 2017. "A Trip to the Alien Planet That Grows America's Mushrooms." *Saveur*, June 2, 2017. Travel section. https://www.saveur.com/mushroom-capital-america-chester-county-pennsylvania-amp.

Alexopoulos, Constantine John. 1962. *Introductory Mycology* second edition. New York: John Wiley and Sons, Inc.

Andrews, Caitlin. 2021. "Maine Legislature Bucks Janet Mills, Police in Voting to Decriminalize Drug Possession." *Bangor Daily News*, June 17, 2021. https://bangordailynews.com/2021/06/17/politics/maine-house-bucks-janet-mills-police-in-vote-to-decriminalize-drug-possession/.

Aouf, Rima Sabina. 2018. "Mushrooms Have the Power to Eat Plastic Say Scientists." *Dezeen*, September 25, 2018. https://www.dezeen.com/2018/09/25/state-of-the-worlds-fungi-report-mushrooms-eat-plastic-kew-gardens/amp/.

Ba, Djibril M. et al. 2021. "Higher Mushroom Consumption is Associated with Lower Risk of Cancer: A Systematic Review and Meta-Analysis of Observational Studies." *Advances in Nutrition* 12, no 5: 1691-1704. https://doi.org/10.1093/advances/nmab015.

Bender, Brian. 2018. "Healthiest Mushrooms: 9 Varieties Ranked by Nutrient Density." October 2, 2018. https://www.intake.health/post/healthiest-mushrooms-9-varieties-ranked-by-nutrient-density.

Beyer, Jennifer. 2017. "A Radical New Approach to Beating Addiction." *Psychology Today*, May 2, 2017. https://www.psychologytoday.com/us/articles/201705/radical-new-approach-beating-addiction.

Black, Jacquelyn G. 2005. *Microbiology Principles and Explorations* sixth edition. Hoboken: John Wiley and Sons Inc.

Bradley, Raymond, et al. 2005. "How Will Global Warming of 2°C Affect Maine?" Climate System Research Center University of Massachusetts, Amherst.
https://www.geo.umass.edu/climate/stateClimateReports/ME_ClimateReport_CSRC.pdf.

British Nutrition Foundation. 2012. "Protein in the Diet." October 2012. www.nutrition.org.uk/media/yh2botxi/protein-in-the-diet_resource.pdf.

Cardwell, Glenn, et al. 2018. "A Review of Mushrooms as a Potential Source of Dietary Vitamin D." *Nutrients* 10, no. 10 (Oct 11, 2018): 1498. https://doi.org/10.3390/nu10101498.

Carluccio, Antonio. 2003. *The Complete Mushroom Book: The Quiet Hunt*. New York: Rizzoli International Publications.

Chang, Shu-Ting, and Philip G. Miles. 2004. *Mushrooms: Cultivation, Nutritional Value, Medicinal Effect, and Environmental Impact* second edition. Boca Raton: CRC Press.

Chang, Shu-Ting, and Solomon, P. Wasser. 2012. "The Role of Culinary-Medicinal Mushrooms on Human Welfare with a Pyramid Model for Human Health." *International Journal of Medicinal Mushrooms* 14, no 2: 95-134. https://doi.org/10.1615/intjmedmushr.v14.i2.10.

Cramer, Claire Z. 2018. "Mushroom Magic." *Portland Monthly*, May, 2018. https://www.portlandmonthly.com/portmag/2018/04/mushroom-magic/.

Crook, Lizzie. 2020. "Circular Union Uses Mushrooms to Create Eco-friendly Mush-Hues Dyes." *Dezeen*, April 29, 2020. https://www.dezeen.com/2020/04/29/circular-union-mush-hues-ventura-projects-vdf/amp/.

Curtis, Abigail. 2017. "Maine Mushroom Growers Tapping Into a Love of Fungi." *Bangor Daily News*, November 25, 2017. https://www.bangordailynews.com/2017/11/25/living/maine-mushroom-growers-tapping-into-a-love-of-fungi/.

Dadachova, Ekaterina, and Arturo Casadevall. 2008. "Ionizing Radiation: How Fungi Cope, Adapt, and Exploit With the Help of Melanin." *Current Opinion in Microbiology* 11, no. 6 (December 2008): 525-31. https://doi.org/10.1016/j.mib.2008.09.013.

Daniel, Jeremy, and Margaret Haberman. 2017. "Clinical Potential of Psilocybin as a Treatment for Mental Health Conditions." *Mental Health Clinician* 7, no. 1 (January): 24-8. https://doi.org/10.9740/mhc.2017.01.024.

De Silva, Dilani D. et al. 2012. "Medicinal Mushrooms in Prevention and Control of Diabetes Mellitus." *Fungal Diversity* 56: 1-29. https://doi.org/10.1007/s13225-012-0187-4.

Devash, Meirav. 2018. "The Benefits of Adding Snow Mushrooms to Your Skin-Care Routine." Yahoo, November 5, 2018. https://www.yahoo.com/amphtml/lifestyle/benefits-adding-snow-mushroom-skin-130000559.html.

Farra, Emily. 2021. "Stella McCartney Introduces her First Garments Made of Mylo, the "Leather" Alternative Grown From Mushrooms." *Vogue*, March 18, 2021. https://vogue.co.uk

Gabriel, Steve. 2015. "Mushrooms Turning a Profit for Forest Farmers in the Northeast." Cornell Small Farms Program, winter 2015. https://smallfarms.cornell.edu/2015/01/12/mushrooms/.

Gebhart, Susan E., and Tobin G. Thomas. 2002. "Nutritive Value of Foods." Agricultural Research Service, USDA. https://www.ars.usda.gov/arsuserfiles/80400525/data/hg72/hg72_2002.pdf.

Graham, Ada, and Frank Graham Jr. 1995. *Kate Furbish and the Flora of Maine*. Gardiner: Tilbury House.

Guggenheim, Alena, et al. 2014. "Immune Modulation from Five Major Mushrooms: Application to Integrative Oncology." *Integrative Medicine* (Encinitas) 13, no. 1 (February): 32-44. https://www.ncbi.nlm.nih.gov/pmc/articles/PMC4684115/.

Hall, Christine, 2022. "Mycoworks, Making Leather From Fungi, Closes $125M to Scale Production." *TechCrunch*. January 13, 2022. https://www.techcrunch.com/2022/01/13/mycoworks-leather-fungi-scale-production/amp/.

Haytowitz, David B. 2006. "Nutrient Content and Nutrient Retention of Selected Mushrooms." USDA Nutrient Data Lab, Beltsville Human Nutrition Research Center, USDA-ARS, Beltsville. MD. http://www.ars.usda.gov/ARSUserFiles/80400525/articles/ift2006 mushroom.pdf.

Hobbs, Christopher. 2020. *Medical Mushrooms: The Essential Guide*. North Adams: Storey Publishing.

Huang, Wen-Chin et al. 2019. "Chinese Herbal Medicine *Ganoderma tsugae* Displays Potential Anti-cancer Efficacy on Metastatic Prostate Cancer

Cells." *International Journal of Molecular Sciences* 20, no. 18 (September): 4418-30. https://doi.org/10.3390/ijms20184418.

Isokauppila, Tero. 2017. *Healing Mushrooms: A Practical and Culinary Guide to Using Mushrooms for Whole Body Health*. New York: Avery.

Kabir, Y. et al. 1987. "Effect of Shiitake (*Lentinus edodes*) and Maitake (*Grifola frondosa*) Mushrooms on Blood Pressure and Plasma Lipids of Spontaneously Hypertensive Rats." *Journal of Nutritional Science and Vitaminology* 33, no. 5 (October): 341-6. https://doi.org/10.3117/jnsv.33.341.PMID:3443885.

Kolundžić, Marina, et al. 2016. "Antibacterial and Cytotoxic Activities of Wild Mushroom *Fomes fomentarius* (L.) Fr., Polyporaceae." *Industrial Crops and Products* 79: 110-5. https://doi.org/10.1016/j.indcrop.2015.10.030.

Knowles, Victoria. 2015. "Say Sayonara to Styrofoam and Hello to Mushroom Materials." Greenbiz. January 9, 2015. https://www.greenbiz.com/article/say-sayonara-styrofoam-and-hello-mushroom materials.

Lee, Kuo-Hsiung, et al. 2012. "Recent Progress of Research on Medicinal Mushrooms, Foods, and Other Herbal Products Used in Traditional Chinese Medicine." *Journal of Traditional and Complementary Medicine* 2, no. 2 (April – June): 84-95. https://www.ncbi.nlm.nih.gov/pmc/articlesPMC3942920/.

Lincoff, Gary. 1981. *National Audubon Society Field Guide to North American Mushrooms*. New York: Alfred A. Knopf.

Mádara Cosmetics. 2020. "Let Your Hair Grow Like Mushrooms." http://www.madaracosmetics.com/en/blog/let-your-hair-grow-like-mushrooms.

Marley, Greg. 2009. *Mushrooms for Health: Medicinal Secrets of Northeastern Fungi*. Rockport: Down East Books.

Marley, Greg. 2010. *Chanterelle Dreams, Amanita Nightmares: The Love, Lore, and Mystique of Mushrooms*. White River Junction: Chelsea Green Publishing Company.

Marley, Greg. 2020. "Mushroom Foraging in Maine and New England, Trends, Favorites and Stories." You Tube video of talk at Camden Memorial Library, Biddeford, Maine, April 16, 2020.

Marley, Greg. 2022. "Foraging for Edible Mushrooms: Embracing a Foolproof Few for Your Area (Developed for New England). You Tube video of talk at McArthur Public Library, Biddeford, Maine, February 3, 2022.

Marley, Greg. 2022. "Integrating Medicinal Mushrooms into Your Life." You Tube video of talk at McArthur Public Library, Biddeford, Maine, March 22, 2022.

Matthews, Allen, et al. 2014. "Log-Based Shiitake Cultivation – SARE Northeast." https:/www.northeast.sare.org/resources/log-based-shiitake-cultivation/.

McKay, Gretchen. 2008. "World's Largest Mushroom Facility Here." *Pittsburg Post-Gazette*, August 28, 2008. https://www.post-gazette.com/life/food/2008/08/28/World-s-largest-mushroom-facility-here/stories/200808280505.

Memorial Sloan Kettering Cancer Center. "Shiitake Mushroom." June 8, 2020.https://www.mskcc.org/pdf/cancer-care/patient-education/herbs/shiitake-mushroom.

Morgan, Genevieve. 2019. "Shroom Nation." *Edible Maine*, September 15, 2019. https://www.ediblemaine.com/editorial-1/Shroom-Nation.

National Cancer Institute. 2019. "Medicinal Mushrooms (PDQ®) – Patient Version." January 17, 2019. https://www.ncbi.nml.nih.gov/books/NBK424937/.

Ostry, Michael, E. et al. 2011. "Field Guide to Common Macrofungi in Eastern Forests and Their Ecosystem Functions." Revised February 2017. United States Forest Service General Technical Reports NRS-79. https://doi.org/10.2737/NRS-GTR-79.

Pace, Giuseppe. 1998. *Mushrooms of the World*. Buffalo: Firefly Books Inc.

Patel, Seema, and Arun Goyal. 2012. "Recent Developments in Mushrooms as Anti-cancer Therapeutics: a Review." *3 Biotechnology* 2, no. 1 (March, 2012): 1-15. https://doi.org/10.1007/s13205-011-0036-2.

PRNewswire. 2021. "Medicinal Mushrooms Market to Grow at a CAGR of 9.15% by 2025." December 10, 2021. https://www.prnewswire.com/news-releases/medicinal-mushrooms-market-to-grow-at-a-cagr-of-9-15-by-2025-health-promoting-benefits-of-medicinal-mushrooms-to-boost-market-17000-technavio-reports-301442077.html.

Quan-Yu et al. 2013. "The Triterpenoids of *Ganoderma tsugae* prevent stress-induced mycocardial injury in mice." *Molecular Nutrition & Food Research* 57, no. 10 (October, 2013): 1892-6. https://doi.org/10.1002/mnfr.201200704.

Roberts, Chris. 2020. "Oregon Legalizes Psilocybin Mushrooms and Decriminalizes all Drugs." *Forbes*, November 4, 2020. https://www.forbes.com/sites/chrisroberts/2020/11/04/oregon-legalizes-psilocybin-mushrooms-and-decriminalizes-all-drugs/amp/.

Rogers, Robert, D. 2015. "Chicken of the Woods - Medicinal Mycology." *Fungi* 8, no. 4 (winter): 23-6. https:/www.academia.edu/20578775/Chicken of the woods Medicinal Mycology.

Rootman, Joseph M. et al. 2021. "Adults who Microdose Psychedelics Report Health Related Motivations and Lower Levels of Anxiety and Depression Compared to Non-microdosers." *Nature Scientific Reports* 11, (November 2021): 22479. https://doi.org/10.1038/s41598-021-01811-4.

Russell, Stephen. 2014. *The Essential Guide to Cultivating Mushrooms*. North Adams: Storey Books.

Sarnacki, Aislinn. 2012. "Foraging for Fungi, from Maine to Mario Land." *Bangor Daily News*, October 3, 2012, updated March 29, 2021. https://bangordailynews.com/2012/10/03/news/foraging-for-fungi-from-maine-to-mario-land-2/.

Sarnacki, Aislinn. 2018. "What You Need to Know About Poisonous Mushrooms Before Foraging." *Bangor Daily News*, September 11, 2018, updated June 29, 2021. https://bangordailynews.com/2018/09/11/homestead/what-you-need-to-know-about-poisonous-mushrooms-before-foraging/.

Schlanger, Zoë. 2021. "The Mushrooms Will Survive Us." *New York Times*, February 7, 2021.

https://www.nytimes.com/2021/02/07style/growing-mushrooms.amp.html.

Sertic, Genevieve. 2016. "Portobello Power: Mushrooms Make for Environmentally Friendly Batteries." *Yale Scientific*, February 3, 2016. https://www.yalescientific.org/2016/02/portobello–power–mushrooms–make–for–environmentally–friendly–batteries/.

Sheldrake, Merlin. 2020. *Entangled Life: How Fungi Make our Worlds, Change our Minds and Shape our Futures*. New York: Penguin Random House.

Sinclair, Amy. 2014. "Indoor Maine Mushroom Farm Harvests 150 Pounds of Fungi Weekly." New England Cable News, April 16, 2014. https://www.necn.com/news/business/_necn_indoor_maine_mushroom_farm_harvests_150_pounds_of_fungi_weekly_necn/1930520/amp.

Skelton, Kathryn. 2022. "Uncle and Nephew Start a Family Mushroom Farm in Auburn." *Sun Journal*, January 27, 2022. https://www.sunjournal.com/2022/01/27/uncle–and–nephew–start–a–family–mushroom–farm/.

Slator William. 2021. "Reishi Mushrooms for Hair Growth: 2021 Guide." June 19, 2021. https://www.hairguard.com/reishi-mushroom/.

Spahr, David, L. 2009. *Edible and Medicinal Mushrooms of New England and Eastern Canada*. Berkeley: North Atlantic Books.

Stamets, Paul. 1993. *Growing Gourmet and Medicinal Mushrooms*. Berkeley: Ten Speed Press.

Stamets, Paul. 2005. *Mycelium Running: How Mushrooms Can Help Save the World*. Berkeley: Ten Speed Press.

Stamets, Paul, ed. 2019. *Fantastic Fungi: How Mushrooms Can Heal, Shift Consciousness and Save the Planet*. San Rafael: Earth Aware.

Stamets, Paul and Jeff S. Chilton. 1983. *The Mushroom Cultivator: A Practical Guide to Growing Mushrooms at Home*. Seattle: Agarikon Press.

Tang, Calyn, et al. 2016. "Golden Needle Mushroom: A Culinary Medicine with Evidence-Based Biological Activities and Health Promoting Properties." *Frontiers in Pharmacology* 7: 474. https://doi.org/:10.3389/fphar.2016.00474.

Teplyakova, Tamara, et al. 2012. "Antiviral Activity of Polyporoid Mushrooms (Higher Basidiomyctes) from Altai Mountains (Russia)." *International Journal of Medicinal Mushrooms* 14, no. 1: 37-45. https://doi.org/:10.16115/intjmedmushr.v14.i1.40. PMID: 22339706.

Therkelsen, Stig Palm, et al. 2016. "Effect of a Medicinal *Agaricus blazei* Murill-based Mushroom Extract, AndoSan™, on Symptoms, Fatigue and Quality of Life in Patients with Ulcerative Colitis in a Randomized Single-Blinded Placebo Controlled Study." *PLOS One* 11, no. 3: e0150191.https://doi.org/:10.1371/journal.pone.0150191.

Tsukagoshi, S., Y. et al. 1984. "Krestin (PSK)." *Cancer Treatment Reviews* 11, no. 2: 131-55. https://doi.org/:10.016/0305-7372(84)90005-7.

University of Maryland. 2021. "US Beekeepers Continue to Report High Colony Loss Rates, No Clear Improvement." *Science Daily*, June 23, 2021. https://www.sciencedaily.com/releases/2021/06/210623193939.html.

Valigra, Lori. 2012. "Mushroom Business Grows from New Technology." Mainebiz, December 24, 2012. https://www.mainebiz.biz/article/mushroom-business-grows-from-new-technology.

Valigra, Lori. 2017. "Beyond Mushroom Soup: Maine Growers Cultivate Gourmet Mushrooms". Mainebiz, July 10, 2017, Focus: Southern Maine. https://www.mainebiz.biz/article/beyond-mushroom-soup-maine-growers-cultivate-gourmet-mushrooms.

Valverde, Maria Elena, et al. 2015. "Edible Mushrooms: Improving Human Health and Promoting Quality Life." *International Journal of Microbiology* January 20, 2015. Article ID 376387. https://doi.org/:10.1155/2015/376387. PMID: 25685150.

Waldman, Gordon. 2019. "What Psilocybin Could Mean for End-of-Life Care." *Psychology Today* July 15, 2019. https://www.psychologytoday.com/us/blog/the-guest-room/201907/what-psilocybin-could-mean-end-life-care/amp.

Ware, Megan. 2019. "What is the Nutritional Value of Mushrooms?" *Medical News Today* November 6, 2019. https://wwww.medicalnewstoday.com/articles/278858.

Whole Foods Market. 2019. "Whole Foods Market Predicts Top 10 Food Trends for 2020." October 21, 2019. https://media.wholefoodsmarket.com/whole-foods-market-predicts-top-10-food-trends-for-2020.

Willis, Katherine, J. 2018. "State of the World's Fungi." Royal Botanic Gardens, Kew. https://stateoftheworldsfungi.org./.

Wolfe, David. 2012. *Chaga: King of Medicinal Mushrooms.* Berkeley: North Atlantic Books.

Wu, Yuanzheng, et al. 2016. "Mushroom Cosmetics: The Present and Future." *Cosmetics* 3, no. 3 (July 8, 2016): 22. https://doi.org/10.3390/cosmetics3030022.

ACKNOWLEDGEMENTS

Huge hugs go out to my artist and writer buddies, Linda Sapienza and Cheryl Blaydon, for their tremendous support, encouragement and suggestions on early drafts of this manuscript. My daughter, Joyce Chagan, also gets a special tribute for help with graphics. Special thanks go to Eliah Thanhauser of North Spore, Candice Hoydon of Oyster Creek Mushroom Company, Aron Gonsalves of Mousam Valley Mushrooms, Suzanne Lametta of Bramble Hill Farm, Justin Wood of Sweetwoods Farm, and staff at Boothbay Harbor and Southport Memorial Libraries for providing information for this project. I am also grateful to Erik Lomen for his fascinating tour of Maine Cap N' Stem's production plant. Many thanks go to forager and chef, Frank Giglio, for providing stories, a couple of recipes and a photo. Plus gratitude is extended to Betsy Bass and Terry Kimball, who kept me posted from spring through fall with wonderful mushroom shots. Photo credits also go to Rita Arnold. Special thanks go to Mariah Wright of Circular Union, for providing details and images of their Mush-Hues project. A shout out goes to Jean Wood, Candice Hoydon of Oyster Creek Mushroom Company and writer Roberta Bailey for sharing recipes. And finally, special thanks go to my publisher, Pat Newell, at North Country Press.

ABOUT THE AUTHOR

Hilary Bartlett was born and raised in postwar Liverpool, England, a predominantly Irish city where markets stocked a dozen varieties of potatoes, rarely mushrooms. Hilary studied fungi as part of her microbiology training and earned her doctorate from University College London.

A summer science fellowship brought Hilary to Boothbay Harbor in 1975 to work at Bigelow Lab. She was supposed to return to London but Maine's rocky coast bewitched her — she never left. Hilary first hunted for wild mushrooms when she came to live in rural Maine. She quit scientific research after her daughter was born and started a home-based art business. Hilary's paintings have been exhibited at galleries in Maine and Santa Fe, New Mexico, some have won awards. She also taught microbiology for eleven years at the University of Maine Augusta.

Her first book, *The Thistle Inn: A Wee Bit of Scotland in Maine*, was published in 2020 by North Country Press.

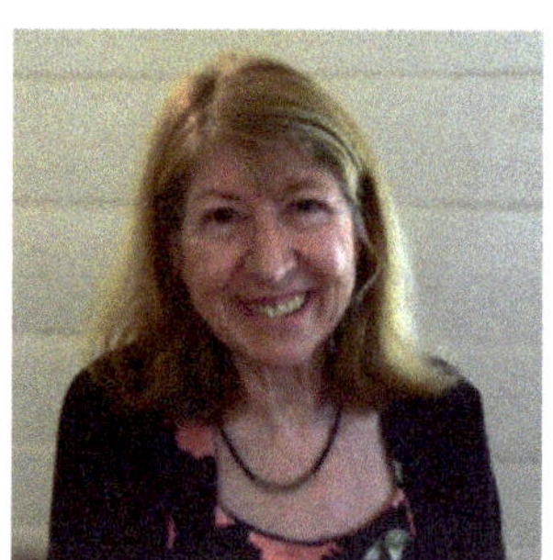

Hilary Bartlett, author. Bob Crink

SUBJECT INDEX

www.ingramcontent.com/pod-product-compliance
Lightning Source LLC
LaVergne TN
LVHW052353100826
845147LV00013B/830

* 9 7 8 1 9 4 3 4 2 4 8 1 8 *